NATUROPATHY
for
LONGEVITY

NATUROPATHY *for* LONGEVITY

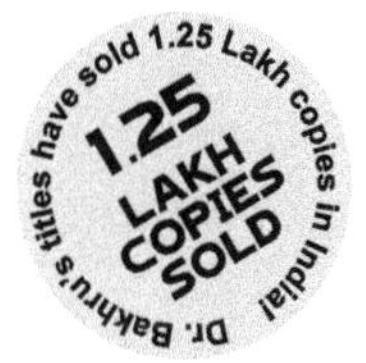

DR. H. K. BAKHRU
NATIONALLY ACCLAIMED NATUROPATH

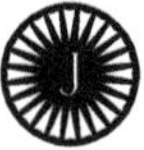

JAICO PUBLISHING HOUSE
Ahmedabad Bangalore Bhopal Bhubaneswar Chennai
Delhi Hyderabad Kolkata Lucknow Mumbai

Published by Jaico Publishing House
A-2 Jash Chambers, 7-A Sir Phirozshah Mehta Road
Fort, Mumbai - 400 001
jaicopub@jaicobooks.com
www.jaicobooks.com

NATUROPATHY FOR LONGEVITY
ISBN 81-7224-629-3

First Jaico Impression: 2000
Tenth Jaico Impression (Reformatted): 2013
Eleventh Jaico Impression: 2014

Printed by

About the Author

DR. H. K. BAKHRU was an expert naturopath and a prolific writer. His well-researched articles on nature cure, health, nutrition and herbs appear regularly in various newspapers and magazines and they bear the stamp of authority.

A diploma holder in naturopathy, all his 13 books on nature cure, nutrition and herbs titled, *A Complete Handbook of Nature Cure*, *Diet Cure for Common Ailments*, *A Handbook of Natural Beauty*, *Nature Cure for Children*, *Naturopathy for Longevity*, *Healing Through Natural Foods*, *Indian Spices and Condiments as Natural Healers*, *Foods That Heal*, *Herbs That Heal*, *Natural Home Remedies for Common Ailments*, *Vitamins that Heal*, *Conquering Diabetes Naturally* and *Conquering Cancer Naturally* have been highly appreciated by the public and repeatedly reprinted. His first-named book was awarded first prize in the category 'Primer on Naturopathy for Healthy Living' by the jury of judges at the 'Book Prize Award' scheme, organized by 'National Institute of Naturopathy', an autonomous body under Government of India, Ministry of Health.

Dr. Bakhru began his career on the Indian Railways, with a first class first postgraduate degree in History from Lucknow University in 1949. He retired in October 1984 as the Chief Public Relations Officer of the Central Railway in Mumbai, having to his credit 35 years of distinguished service in the Public Relations organisations of the Indian Railways and the Railway Board.

An associate member of the All India Alternative Medical Practitioner's Association and a member of the Nature Cure Practitioners' Guild in Mumbai, Dr. Bakhru had extensively studied herbs and natural methods of treating diseases. He had been honoured with 'Lifetime Achievement Award', 'Gem of Alternative Medicines' award and a gold medal in Diet Therapy by the Indian Board of Alternative Medicines, Kolkata, in recognition of his dedication and outstanding contributions in the field of Alternative Medicines. The Board, which is affiliated with the Open International University for Complementary Medicines, established under World Health Organisation and recognised by the United Nations Peace University, had also appointed him as its Honorary Advisor. Dr. Bakhru had also been honoured by Nature Cure Practitioners' Guild, Mumbai with Nature Cure Appreciation Award for his services to Naturopathy.

Dr. Bakhru was the founder of a registered Public Charitable Trust, known as D.H. Bakhru Foundation, to help the poor and needy.

Preface

How can one keep fit in old age and live longer? This book explains at some length the various factors which contribute to health and fitness, and impart energy and vitality in old age. It also deals with diseases commonly prevalent in the elderly and prescribes time-tested nature cure methods for their treatment.

Fitness, however, is a relative term. It is difficult to find a person with perfect health these days. Faced with the growing complexities of modern life and the resultant crises — living in polluted environments and consuming denatured, refined foods — one has to make strenuous efforts today to keep himself fit, especially in old age. The task is even more difficult for elderly people. Dr. Bakhru had suffered immensely from a very early age, mainly due to the shortcomings of the modern medical system. A brief case history will drive home the point.

His troubles began at 16, when he contracted dry pleurisy and typhoid fever simultaneously. Having run their course for about 45 days, both the ailments made him very weak. His recovery was gradual but not complete, as he soon developed heartburn and breathing trouble.

At 28, came the worst crisis, when he suffered a stroke in the early hours of an exceptionally hot day, following severe heartburn throughout the night. The stroke made the left side of his body extremely heavy and weak. The attending physician, suspecting a brain tumour, referred his case to a well known neurosurgeon. For some two months, he was subjected to drastic tests which failed to locate the imaginary brain tumour. The harrowing experience left him a complete wreck.

Add to it a barium meal examination revealed chronic duodenal ulcer. The various drugs prescribed for this disease and the continuing weakness and heaviness of his left side made his condition worse. He endured this for three years, until the pain and heaviness of his left side was miraculously cured by an astrologer. But nothing could rid him of the heartburn, abdominal pain and occasional stomach upsets. A barium meal examination, done when he was 39, also revealed hiatus hernia with peptic esophageal ulcers.

To add to all these, at 45, an eminent heart specialist declared him as a heart patient. The heavy drugging and dieting that ensued completely ruined his health and resulted in insomnia and a weight loss of 15 kg. Two years later, a second opinion from a renowned heart specialist, revealed there was no evidence, whatsoever, of heart trouble. He, however, confirmed the presence of duodenal ulcer and hiatus hernia. Then came a host of diseases in quick succession — cervical spondylitis, myalgia, backache and prostate enlargement. In treating all these diseases, the modern medical system failed miserably.

Finding no conventional allopathic cure or treatment for his ailments, rather late in the day, at the age of 55, he made a determined bid to do away with all the medicines and take recourse to natural methods. He made a deep study of nature cure, consulted expert naturopaths, made drastic changes in his diet and lifestyle, and started following the laws of nature rigidly. Though he made no claims to cure all ailments, he managed to control them substantially.

The two dominant factors in the maintenance of his health

were firm determination to keep fit and to forget that he suffered from any serious medical problem.

The various measures adopted in respect of the first factor included consumption of natural, unrefined foods as far as possible, regular practice of yogasanas and other physical exercises, especially walking, occasional use of hydrotherapy, avoidance of late hours and following other laws of nature.

With regard to the second factor, he kept himself fully occupied so that all thoughts about his illness were diverted. he devoted his time popularising nature cure by writing articles and books on the subject and offering personal and postal advice to those who seeked his help in solving their health problems.

He did all this, despite being a handicapped person. He suffered from extremely low vision due to degeneration of retina of both the eyes. His right eye's vision was negligible and he could read typed letters only with the help of a high-powered magnifying glass fitted in the left side of the spectacles. He earnestly hoped that all his painstaking efforts would serve as an inspiration to his fellow senior citizens to keep themselves occupied with constructive activities irrespective of the difficulties they faced.

Contents

Section II: Nervous System and Mental Disorders

Section III: Low Vision

Section IV: Cardiovascular System Disorder

Section V: Respiratory System Disorders

Section VI: Diseases of the Gastrointestinal System

Section VII: Musculo-Skeleton System Disorders

Section VIII: Diseases of the Kidney and Urinary System

Section IX: Diseases of the Endocrine System

Section X: Other Diseases

Appendices

Introduction
Ageing Process and Longevity

Individuals age at different rates. In fact, even within one person, organs and organ systems show different rates of decline. However, based on recent studies on ageing, some general features regarding ageing are described herein, which may not apply to all people.

The heart grows slightly larger with age. Maximal oxygen consumption during exercise declines in men by about 10 per cent with each decade of adult life and in women by about 7.5 per cent. However, cardiac output stays nearly the same because the heart pumps more efficiently. There is a gradual loss of elastic tissue in lungs of an ageing person. The walls of the air cells tend to break down and some of the elastic tissue is replaced by fibrous tissue. Both these processes reduce the capacity of the lungs to extract oxygen from air. The maximum breathing capacity of lungs also declines by about 40 per cent between the ages of 20 and 70.

The brain loses some cells (neurons) and others become damaged. However, it adapts by increasing the number of connections between cells-synapses and by regrowing the branchlike extensions, dendrites and axons, that carry messages in the brain.

The kidneys gradually become less efficient at extracting morbid matter from the blood. Bladder capacity declines. Urinary incontinence results from tissue atrophy. This can, however, be managed through exercise and behavioural techniques.

From the forties onwards, wear and tear in the cartilages of major joints like knees and hips make for some stiffness of the limbs after prolonged sitting. This may also be noticed in the back of the neck due to some arthritic process in the bones of the spine. Without exercise, estimated muscle mass declines by 22 per cent for woman and 23 per cent for men between the ages of 30 and 70. Exercise can prevent this loss.

A subjective marker, particularly noticeable in older persons, is a change in the ability to read small prints. In the over 40s, the elasticity of the lens in the eyes is reduced, which alters the ability to focus clearly. The defect is corrected by suitable reading glasses.

In women, the most distinctive feature of ageing is the onset of menopause. In physical terms, it refers to the cessation of the monthly period because the ovaries shut down, commonly in the mid or late forties. Menopause can occur prematurely in some women due to wrong feeding and stress. The resultant physical effects include loss of skin sheen, external changes in the breasts which may be reduced in size and firmness, and in the external genitals and internal genital linings.

The various changes of ageing may prove troublesome for the person who experiences them in proportion to their degree and rapidity of onset. It is, however, possible to achieve longevity and its associated delay in natural changes of ageing through nutritional practice and other natural methods.

Longevity: According to Dr. Edward Henderson, past president of the American geriatric society, the age of one hundred is a realistic and conceivable goal. Dr. Thomas Gardiner, one of the founders of the National Foundation for Anti-ageing Research and noted for his research studies with vitamins, believes that we have not even approached the normal span of years. He claims that most ageing is premature, and that body organs are designed to last six to seven times as long as it usually takes the average person to reach maturity. He believes that we could double the life span. It means staying young longer.

The American Medical Association on Ageing has outlined a do-it-yourself check list of how to live longer and better. The list includes a balanced diet, regular elimination of waste products, adequate rest of both mind and body, pursuit of interesting and specific recreational activities, a sense of humour, avoidance of excessive emotional tension, mutual loyalty of friends and family, pride in a job, participation in community affairs and continued expansion of knowledge, wisdom and experience. It will be worthwhile for the elderly to follow these guidelines.

A number of studies have been conducted on the life habits of people in the age group "100 plus." Essentially, the common important factors, contributing to their health and longevity were found to be: adequate rest, retiring to bed early, with a short nap or rest in the afternoon; freedom from tension, stress and worry; daily physical exercise, particularly walking; regularity of daily habits; moderation in all things; a generally placid yet energetic disposition.

Dr. Cecila Hurwich, who has done a longitudinal study on "Vital Women in their 70s, 80s and 90s" and was awarded a PhD in her 70s, has discovered that older people who enjoy life share five characteristics. These are: (i) they find life meaningful, (ii) they are optimistic, (iii) have friends of all ages, (iv) continue to grow and (v) consider spirituality important.

United Nations Principles for Older Persons

To add life to the years that have been added to life The General Assembly, Appreciating the contribution that older persons make to their societies.

Recognizing that, in the Charter of the United Nations, the peoples of the United Nations declare, inter alia, their determination to reaffirm faith in fundamental human rights, in the dignity and worth of the human person, in the equal rights of men and women, and of nations large and small; and to promote social progress and better standards of life in larger freedom.

Noting the elaboration of those rights in the Universal Declaration of Human Rights (General Assembly resolution 217 A(III) of 10 December 1948), the International Convention on Economic, Social and Cultural Rights and the International Convention on Civil and Political Rights (General Assembly resolution 2200 A(XXI), annex, of 16 December 1966) and other declarations to ensure the application of universal standards to particular groups,

In Pursuance of the International Plan of Action on Ageing adopted by the World Assembly on Ageing and endorsed by the

General Assembly in its resolution 37/51 of 3 December 1982 Appreciating the tremendous diversity in the situation of older persons, not only between countries but within countries and between individuals, which requires a variety of policy responses, AWARE that in all countries, individual are reaching an advanced age in greater number and in better health than ever before.

Aware of the scientific research disproving many stereotypes about inevitable and irreversible declines with age, Convinced that in a world characterised by an increasing number and proportion of older persons, opportunities must be provided for willing and capable older persons to participate and contribute to the ongoing activities of society.

Mindful that the strains on family life in both developed and developing countries require support for those providing care to frail older persons.

Bearing in mind the standards already set by the International Plan of Action on Ageing and the conventions, recommendations and resolution of the International Labour Organisation, the World Health Organisation and other United Nations entities,

Encourages Governments to incorporate the following principles into their national programmes whenever possible:

Independence

(1) Older persons should have access to adequate food, water, shelter, clothing and health care through the provision of income, family and community support and self-help.

(2) Older persons should have the opportunity to work or to have access to other income-generating opportunities.

(3) Older persons should be able to participate in determining when and at what pace withdrawal from the labour force takes place.

(4) Older persons should have access to appropriate educational and training programmes.

(5) Older persons should be able to live in environments that are safe and adaptable to personal preferences and changing capacities.

(6) Older persons should be able to reside at home for as long as possible.

Participation

(7) Older persons should remain integrated in society, should participate actively in the formulation and implementation of policies that directly affect their well-being and should share their knowledge and skills with younger generations.

(8) Older persons should be able to seek and develop opportunities for service to the community and to serve as volunteers in positions appropriate to their interests and capabilities.

(9) Older persons should be able to form movements or associations of older persons.

Care

(10) Older persons should benefit from family and community care and protection in accordance with each society's system of cultural values.

(11) Older persons should have access to health care to help them to maintain or regain the optimum level of physical, mental and emotional well-being and to prevent or delay the onset of illness.

(12) Older persons should have access to social and legal services to enhance their autonomy, protection and care.

(13) Older persons should be able to utilize appropriate levels of institutional care providing protection, rehabilitation and social and mental stimulation in a humane and secure environment.

(14) Older persons should be able to enjoy human rights and fundamental freedoms when residing in any shelter, care or treatment facility, including full respect for their dignity, beliefs, needs privacy and for the right to make decisions about their care and quality of life.

Self-fulfillment

(15) Older persons should be able to pursue opportunities for the full development of their potential.

(16) Older persons should have access to the educational, cultural, spiritual and recreational resources of society.

Dignity

(17) Older persons should be able to live in dignity and security and to be free of exploitation and physical or mental abuse.

(18) Older persons should be treated fairly regardless of age, gender, racial or ethnic background, disability or other status, and to be valued independently of their economic contributions."

About the Author

DR. H. K. BAKHRU was an expert naturopath and a prolific writer. His well-researched articles on nature cure, health, nutrition and herbs appear regularly in various newspapers and magazines and they bear the stamp of authority.

A diploma holder in naturopathy, all his 13 books on nature cure, nutrition and herbs titled, *A Complete Handbook of Nature Cure, Diet Cure for Common Ailments, A Handbook of Natural Beauty, Nature Cure for Children, Naturopathy for Longevity, Healing Through Natural Foods, Indian Spices and Condiments as Natural Healers, Foods That Heal, Herbs That Heal, Natural Home Remedies for Common Ailments, Vitamins that Heal, Conquering Diabetes Naturally* and *Conquering Cancer Naturally* have been highly appreciated by the public and repeatedly reprinted. His first-named book was awarded first prize in the category 'Primer on Naturopathy for Healthy Living' by the jury of judges at the 'Book Prize Award' scheme, organized by 'National Institute of Naturopathy', an autonomous body under Government of India, Ministry of Health.

Dr. Bakhru began his career on the Indian Railways, with a first class first postgraduate degree in History from Lucknow University in 1949. He retired in October 1984 as the Chief Public Relations Officer of the Central Railway in Mumbai, having to his credit 35 years of distinguished service in the Public Relations organisations of the Indian Railways and the Railway Board.

An associate member of the All India Alternative Medical Practitioner's Association and a member of the Nature Cure Practitioners' Guild in Mumbai, Dr. Bakhru had extensively studied herbs and natural methods of treating diseases. He had been honoured with 'Lifetime Achievement Award', 'Gem of Alternative Medicines' award and a gold medal in Diet Therapy by the Indian Board of Alternative Medicines, Kolkata, in recognition of his dedication and outstanding contributions in the field of Alternative Medicines. The Board, which is affiliated with the Open International University for Complementary Medicines, established under World Health Organisation and recognised by the United Nations Peace University, had also appointed him as its Honorary Advisor. Dr. Bakhru had also been honoured by Nature Cure Practitioners' Guild, Mumbai with Nature Cure Appreciation Award for his services to Naturopathy.

Dr. Bakhru was the founder of a registered Public Charitable Trust, known as D.H. Bakhru Foundation, to help the poor and needy.

Preface

How can one keep fit in old age and live longer? This book explains at some length the various factors which contribute to health and fitness, and impart energy and vitality in old age. It also deals with diseases commonly prevalent in the elderly and prescribes time-tested nature cure methods for their treatment.

Fitness, however, is a relative term. It is difficult to find a person with perfect health these days. Faced with the growing complexities of modern life and the resultant crises — living in polluted environments and consuming denatured, refined foods — one has to make strenuous efforts today to keep himself fit, especially in old age. The task is even more difficult for elderly people. Dr. Bakhru had suffered immensely from a very early age, mainly due to the shortcomings of the modern medical system. A brief case history will drive home the point.

His troubles began at 16, when he contracted dry pleurisy and typhoid fever simultaneously. Having run their course for about 45 days, both the ailments made him very weak. His recovery was gradual but not complete, as he soon developed heartburn and breathing trouble.

At 28, came the worst crisis, when he suffered a stroke in the early hours of an exceptionally hot day, following severe heartburn throughout the night. The stroke made the left side of his body extremely heavy and weak. The attending physician, suspecting a brain tumour, referred his case to a well known neurosurgeon. For some two months, he was subjected to drastic tests which failed to locate the imaginary brain tumour. The harrowing experience left him a complete wreck.

Add to it a barium meal examination revealed chronic duodenal ulcer. The various drugs prescribed for this disease and the continuing weakness and heaviness of his left side made his condition worse. He endured this for three years, until the pain and heaviness of his left side was miraculously cured by an astrologer. But nothing could rid him of the heartburn, abdominal pain and occasional stomach upsets. A barium meal examination, done when he was 39, also revealed hiatus hernia with peptic esophageal ulcers.

To add to all these, at 45, an eminent heart specialist declared him as a heart patient. The heavy drugging and dieting that ensued completely ruined his health and resulted in insomnia and a weight loss of 15 kg. Two years later, a second opinion from a renowned heart specialist, revealed there was no evidence, whatsoever, of heart trouble. He, however, confirmed the presence of duodenal ulcer and hiatus hernia. Then came a host of diseases in quick succession — cervical spondylitis, myalgia, backache and prostate enlargement. In treating all these diseases, the modern medical system failed miserably.

Finding no conventional allopathic cure or treatment for his ailments, rather late in the day, at the age of 55, he made a determined bid to do away with all the medicines and take recourse to natural methods. He made a deep study of nature cure, consulted expert naturopaths, made drastic changes in his diet and lifestyle, and started following the laws of nature rigidly. Though he made no claims to cure all ailments, he managed to control them substantially.

The two dominant factors in the maintenance of his health

were firm determination to keep fit and to forget that he suffered from any serious medical problem.

The various measures adopted in respect of the first factor included consumption of natural, unrefined foods as far as possible, regular practice of yogasanas and other physical exercises, especially walking, occasional use of hydrotherapy, avoidance of late hours and following other laws of nature.

With regard to the second factor, he kept himself fully occupied so that all thoughts about his illness were diverted. he devoted his time popularising nature cure by writing articles and books on the subject and offering personal and postal advice to those who seeked his help in solving their health problems.

He did all this, despite being a handicapped person. He suffered from extremely low vision due to degeneration of retina of both the eyes. His right eye's vision was negligible and he could read typed letters only with the help of a high-powered magnifying glass fitted in the left side of the spectacles. He earnestly hoped that all his painstaking efforts would serve as an inspiration to his fellow senior citizens to keep themselves occupied with constructive activities irrespective of the difficulties they faced.

Contents

Section II: Nervous System and Mental Disorders

Section III: Low Vision

Section IV: Cardiovascular System Disorder

Section V: Respiratory System Disorders

Section VI: Diseases of the Gastrointestinal System

Section VII: Musculo-Skeleton System Disorders

Section VIII: Diseases of the Kidney and Urinary System

Section IX: Diseases of the Endocrine System

Section X: Other Diseases

Appendices

Introduction
Ageing Process and Longevity

Individuals age at different rates. In fact, even within one person, organs and organ systems show different rates of decline. However, based on recent studies on ageing, some general features regarding ageing are described herein, which may not apply to all people.

The heart grows slightly larger with age. Maximal oxygen consumption during exercise declines in men by about 10 per cent with each decade of adult life and in women by about 7.5 per cent. However, cardiac output stays nearly the same because the heart pumps more efficiently. There is a gradual loss of elastic tissue in lungs of an ageing person. The walls of the air cells tend to break down and some of the elastic tissue is replaced by fibrous tissue. Both these processes reduce the capacity of the lungs to extract oxygen from air. The maximum breathing capacity of lungs also declines by about 40 per cent between the ages of 20 and 70.

The brain loses some cells (neurons) and others become damaged. However, it adapts by increasing the number of connections between cells-synapses and by regrowing the branchlike extensions, dendrites and axons, that carry messages in the brain.

The kidneys gradually become less efficient at extracting morbid matter from the blood. Bladder capacity declines. Urinary incontinence results from tissue atrophy. This can, however, be managed through exercise and behavioural techniques.

From the forties onwards, wear and tear in the cartilages of major joints like knees and hips make for some stiffness of the limbs after prolonged sitting. This may also be noticed in the back of the neck due to some arthritic process in the bones of the spine. Without exercise, estimated muscle mass declines by 22 per cent for woman and 23 per cent for men between the ages of 30 and 70. Exercise can prevent this loss.

A subjective marker, particularly noticeable in older persons, is a change in the ability to read small prints. In the over 40s, the elasticity of the lens in the eyes is reduced, which alters the ability to focus clearly. The defect is corrected by suitable reading glasses.

In women, the most distinctive feature of ageing is the onset of menopause. In physical terms, it refers to the cessation of the monthly period because the ovaries shut down, commonly in the mid or late forties. Menopause can occur prematurely in some women due to wrong feeding and stress. The resultant physical effects include loss of skin sheen, external changes in the breasts which may be reduced in size and firmness, and in the external genitals and internal genital linings.

The various changes of ageing may prove troublesome for the person who experiences them in proportion to their degree and rapidity of onset. It is, however, possible to achieve longevity and its associated delay in natural changes of ageing through nutritional practice and other natural methods.

Longevity: According to Dr. Edward Henderson, past president of the American geriatric society, the age of one hundred is a realistic and conceivable goal. Dr. Thomas Gardiner, one of the founders of the National Foundation for Anti-ageing Research and noted for his research studies with vitamins, believes that we have not even approached the normal span of years. He claims that most ageing is premature, and that body organs are designed to last six to seven times as long as it usually takes the average person to reach maturity. He believes that we could double the life span. It means staying young longer.

The American Medical Association on Ageing has outlined a do-it-yourself check list of how to live longer and better. The list includes a balanced diet, regular elimination of waste products, adequate rest of both mind and body, pursuit of interesting and specific recreational activities, a sense of humour, avoidance of excessive emotional tension, mutual loyalty of friends and family, pride in a job, participation in community affairs and continued expansion of knowledge, wisdom and experience. It will be worthwhile for the elderly to follow these guidelines.

A number of studies have been conducted on the life habits of people in the age group "100 plus." Essentially, the common important factors, contributing to their health and longevity were found to be: adequate rest, retiring to bed early, with a short nap or rest in the afternoon; freedom from tension, stress and worry; daily physical exercise, particularly walking; regularity of daily habits; moderation in all things; a generally placid yet energetic disposition.

Dr. Cecila Hurwich, who has done a longitudinal study on "Vital Women in their 70s, 80s and 90s" and was awarded a PhD in her 70s, has discovered that older people who enjoy life share five characteristics. These are: (i) they find life meaningful, (ii) they are optimistic, (iii) have friends of all ages, (iv) continue to grow and (v) consider spirituality important.

United Nations Principles for Older Persons

To add life to the years that have been added to life The General Assembly, Appreciating the contribution that older persons make to their societies.

Recognizing that, in the Charter of the United Nations, the peoples of the United Nations declare, inter alia, their determination to reaffirm faith in fundamental human rights, in the dignity and worth of the human person, in the equal rights of men and women, and of nations large and small; and to promote social progress and better standards of life in larger freedom.

Noting the elaboration of those rights in the Universal Declaration of Human Rights (General Assembly resolution 217 A(III) of 10 December 1948), the International Convention on Economic, Social and Cultural Rights and the International Convention on Civil and Political Rights (General Assembly resolution 2200 A(XXI), annex, of 16 December 1966) and other declarations to ensure the application of universal standards to particular groups,

In Pursuance of the International Plan of Action on Ageing adopted by the World Assembly on Ageing and endorsed by the

General Assembly in its resolution 37/51 of 3 December 1982 Appreciating the tremendous diversity in the situation of older persons, not only between countries but within countries and between individuals, which requires a variety of policy responses, AWARE that in all countries, individual are reaching an advanced age in greater number and in better health than ever before.

Aware of the scientific research disproving many stereotypes about inevitable and irreversible declines with age, Convinced that in a world characterised by an increasing number and proportion of older persons, opportunities must be provided for willing and capable older persons to participate and contribute to the ongoing activities of society.

Mindful that the strains on family life in both developed and developing countries require support for those providing care to frail older persons.

Bearing in mind the standards already set by the International Plan of Action on Ageing and the conventions, recommendations and resolution of the International Labour Organisation, the World Health Organisation and other United Nations entities,

Encourages Governments to incorporate the following principles into their national programmes whenever possible:

Independence

(1) Older persons should have access to adequate food, water, shelter, clothing and health care through the provision of income, family and community support and self-help.

(2) Older persons should have the opportunity to work or to have access to other income-generating opportunities.

(3) Older persons should be able to participate in determining when and at what pace withdrawal from the labour force takes place.

(4) Older persons should have access to appropriate educational and training programmes.

(5) Older persons should be able to live in environments that are safe and adaptable to personal preferences and changing capacities.

(6) Older persons should be able to reside at home for as long as possible.

Participation

(7) Older persons should remain integrated in society, should participate actively in the formulation and implementation of policies that directly affect their well-being and should share their knowledge and skills with younger generations.

(8) Older persons should be able to seek and develop opportunities for service to the community and to serve as volunteers in positions appropriate to their interests and capabilities.

(9) Older persons should be able to form movements or associations of older persons.

Care

(10) Older persons should benefit from family and community care and protection in accordance with each society's system of cultural values.

(11) Older persons should have access to health care to help them to maintain or regain the optimum level of physical, mental and emotional well-being and to prevent or delay the onset of illness.

(12) Older persons should have access to social and legal services to enhance their autonomy, protection and care.

(13) Older persons should be able to utilize appropriate levels of institutional care providing protection, rehabilitation and social and mental stimulation in a humane and secure environment.

(14) Older persons should be able to enjoy human rights and fundamental freedoms when residing in any shelter, care or treatment facility, including full respect for their dignity, beliefs, needs privacy and for the right to make decisions about their care and quality of life.

Self-fulfillment

(15) Older persons should be able to pursue opportunities for the full development of their potential.

(16) Older persons should have access to the educational, cultural, spiritual and recreational resources of society.

Dignity

(17) Older persons should be able to live in dignity and security and to be free of exploitation and physical or mental abuse.

(18) Older persons should be treated fairly regardless of age, gender, racial or ethnic background, disability or other status, and to be valued independently of their economic contributions."

SECTION I

GENERAL ASPECTS

CHAPTER 1

How to Stay Young Longer

There is a general belief that the ageing process automatically results in poor health, loss of functions, slower mental faculties and development of such frightening diseases as arthritis, cataract and heart attacks. This has been disproved by recent researches on ageing. These findings have shown that longevity with more vigorous living can be achieved through nutritional practice and other natural methods.

Health, however, is a many-sided affair. There is physical health and spiritual health. Radiant, total health means health in all these areas. It also implies the absence of disease in any of these areas. It is a positive condition. There are three most important factors which determine the condition of our bodies and often the lengths of our lives. These are nutrition, activity and mental outlook. How these three factors can help a person to ward off diseases and stay young longer are discussed herein in brief:

Nutrition

Nutrition is the most important of the various factors contributing to good health and longevity. It is the basis of any programme designed to help a person stay young longer. The entire body from heart to brain, from cells and tissues to bloodstream, depends for their survival upon the food we eat.

Dr. Hans Selye, famous for his research on stress, believes that ageing may be caused partly by accumulation of waste products, which prevents the body cells from receiving their proper nourishment. There are certain foods which lead to this condition and cause clogging up of the body's machinery. They starve the various organs of the body of vital nutrients. This can be prevented by proper nutrition and by avoiding harmful foods that hasten ageing. Ideally, a diet should supply the nutritional needs of all the parts of the body, besides normal requirements. It should also leave a margin of safety to allow for inadequate absorption in cases of illness and deficiencies.

Many research studies have been conducted over the last decade to explore nutrition in ageing. These studies have shown that excessive calorie intake for a long period accelerates the age-related decline as seen in physiological dysfunctions. Experiments with animals have proved that calorie restriction increases the life span. The well recognised anti-ageing actions of calorie restriction are to prevent age-related functional deterioration, retard the progress of age-related disease and thereby prolong both mean and maximum life span.

Antioxidants also play a vital role in delaying ageing process. A 1993 Harvard University study of 40,000 male health professionals found that those who took Vitamin E had a 37 per cent lower rate of heart disease. In older people, Vitamin E dramatically boosts the immune system. Many doctors in the United States, however, recommend 100 to 400 international units of Vitamin E a day, 500 to 1,000 mgs of Vitamin C, and 15 to 25 mgs of beta carotene everyday. Good natural sources of antioxidants are spinach, carrots, broccoli, oranges, bananas, sweet potatoes, almonds and peanut butter.

Activity

Next to nutrition, activity is the most important factor contributing to health and longevity. Activity involves not only the physical activity to keep the muscles firm and strong, but also the activity of the mind to keep the thought processes and emotions flexible. Nothing is more ageing than boredom and idleness. Lazy people do not live long. Many and varied interests should be developed so as to keep oneself fully occupied.

The mind is at its best when occupied usefully and constructively. One should not worry about using up one's brain. In fact, not using it can lead to mental deterioration. All evidence points to the fact that the brain is a sturdy organ, capable of giving efficient service for a hundred years or more. The mind should always therefore be kept busy with subjects that are absorbing, preferably those that present a challenge to stimulate and develop thought.

Mental Outlook

The ageing process can be speeded up or retarded by the way we habitually look at life. This factor is of great importance, especially after a person reaches the age of 40. It is said that a person is as young as he feels. Bernard Baruch, when he was past 80, said, "I always think of old age as being 15 years older than I am".

There is evidence that worry kills more people than work. Joe D. Nichols, MD, wrote: "There are six chief causes of disease, namely, emotional, nutritional, poisons, infections, accidents and inherited. The greatest cause of disease without doubt, is emotional. Worry, fear, anxiety, hate, envy and jealousy, all these are the great killers."

The most important step towards healthy old age is thus a change in attitude. It should be understood that there is nothing about old age which necessitates poor health. There are probably no diseases caused by old age. Diseases associated with old age are usually the ones which take decades to develop and are caused by persistent strain on an organ or faulty nutrition. The body does not wear out but is literally degenerated by a deficient diet with disastrous results.

All living persons aspire to prolong their lives. For this purpose, they are deeply interested in maintaining their physical strength, mental vigour and their zest for living. It is not a difficult task as explained in the preceding paragraphs. All they have to do is to acquire knowledge about the right foods to eat, the most effective ways of exercising and methods for preserving the body's natural energies to put this knowledge into practice. The chapters that follow in this book offer this knowledge and prescribe time-tested natural methods for treating specific diseases commonly prevalent in the elderly.

CHAPTER 2

Nutrition for Vigour and Vitality in Old Age

Nutrition plays a vital role in the maintenance of good health and in the prevention and treatment of disease. There is hardly any evidence to suggest that structural or functional age-related changes, have much of an impact on the ability to eat and digest food. Most old people are capable of reasonably effective mastication. Even where masticatory ability is poor, there is little evidence that overall nutrition suffers. Although atrophic gastritis and abnormalities of the small bowel mucosa become more common with advancing age, these changes do not cause any significant impairment of the ability to absorb food in general.

A well-balanced correct diet for the elderly should take into account two important factors. Firstly, it should supply all the essential nutrients needed by the body so as to prevent deficiency diseases. Secondly, it should help maintain the normal body chemistry which is approximately 20 per cent acid and 80 per cent alkaline. It has been found that a diet which contains liberal quantities of (i) seeds, nuts and grains, (ii) vegetables and (iii) fruits, would provide adequate amounts of all the essential nutrients. These foods have, therefore, been aptly called basis food groups and the diet containing these foods, as optimum diet for vigour and vitality.

Seeds, nuts and grains are the most important and the most potent of all foods. They contain the germ, the reproductive power which is of vital importance for the health of human beings. Seeds, nuts and grains are also excellent natural sources of essential unsaturated fatty acids necessary for health. They are also good sources of lecithin and most of the B Vitamins and the best natural sources of Vitamin C, which is perhaps the most important vitamin for the preservation of health in old age and prevention of premature ageing.

Vegetables are an extremely rich source of minerals, enzymes and vitamins. Faulty cooking and prolonged careless storage, however, destroy these valuable nutrients. Most vegetables are, therefore, best consumed in their natural raw state in the form of salads. To prevent loss of nutrients in vegetables, it would be advisable to steam or boil vegetables in their juices on a slow fire and the water of cooking liquid should not be drained off.

Like vegetables, fruits are excellent sources of minerals, vitamins and enzymes. They are easily digested and exercise a cleansing effect on the blood and digestive tract. They contain high alkalising properties, a high percentage of water and a low percentage of proteins and fats. Fruits are at their best when eaten in the raw and ripe states.

These three basic health-building foods should be supplemented with certain special protective foods such as milk, vegetable oils and honey. Milk is considered as "Nature's most nearly perfect food." The best way to take milk is in its soured form, that is, yogurt, buttermilk and cottage cheese. Soured milk is superior to sweet milk as it is in a predigested form and more easily assimilated. High quality unrefined vegetable oils should be added to the diet. They are rich in unsaturated fatty acids, Vitamin C and F and lecithin. The average daily amount should not exceed two tablespoons. Honey, too, is an ideal food. It helps increase calcium retention in the system, prevents nutritional anaemia, besides being beneficial in kidney and liver disorders, colds and poor circulation. It is one of the finest energy-giving foods.

The diet of the elderly should be so arranged as to provide 80 per cent of alkaline forming foods such as ripe fruits, tubers, leafy and root vegetables, and 20 per cent acid forming foods such as bread, cereals and meats so as to maintain proper acid-alkaline balance in the body. Eating sensibly in this manner will ensure the necessary alkalinity of the blood, which will keep the body in perfect health in old age. The chart showing the common foods with acid and alkaline ash is given in the appendix.

Errors in nutrition either by overfeeding or underfeeding result in premature ageing. One of the important characteristics of really old and healthy people is moderation in all matters. The diet should contain all the required ingredients for maintaining the health without taxing the gastrointestinal system. The general rules pertaining to diet for the attainment of healthy old age are as follows:

(i) Foods should be eaten slowly and chewed thoroughly as digestion begins in the mouth.
(ii) Foods which are very hot or very cold should be avoided.
(iii) Any drink taken with meals or up to an hour later interferes with the digestion.
(iv) Simple meals without sauces are easier to digest.
(v) Fried and roasted foods are difficult to digest and should, therefore, be taken in small quantities.
(vi) The ideal diet for the elderly should consist of 10 per cent protein, 20 per cent carbohydrates, 5 per cent fats and 65 per cent fruits and vegetables.

Two nutritional disasters, which undermine the health and vigour, are white flour and white sugar and all articles of food which have both or one of these items as main ingredients. This covers a wide range of food products such as breads, cakes, biscuits, sweets, jams and soft drinks. Harmful effects of such foods have been discussed in Chapter 5.

Refined carbohydrates and saturated fats constitute a threat to real nutrition. They are made worse because of toxic food additives, pesticides, growth stimulants, preservatives and colouring agents. Their continued use leads to decline in health and resistance to disease as the years progress. This eventually results in crippling diseases which do not kill. Such crippling diseases, especially various forms of arthritis, however, limit life and make old age difficult.

The elderly should also observe the rules of food combining, which is a simple, scientifically based system of selecting foods, from among many different types, which are compatible. This will facilitate easy and efficient digestion and ensure after-meal comfort. It is the combining of many varieties and incompatible foods at a meal that causes 90 per cent of digestive disorders.

The most important rule for combining foods is to avoid mixing protein and carbohydrates concentrated foods and to avoid mixing carbohydrates and acid fruits in the same meal. Protein foods are best digested when eaten with fresh vegetable salad. They also combine very well with sub-acid fruits. Other important rules for food combining are to avoid mixing proteins and fats and mixing carbohydrates and acid fruits at the same meal. In a nutshell, starches, fats, green vegetables and sugars may be eaten together as they require either an alkaline or neutral medium for their digestion. Similarly, proteins, green vegetables and acid fruits, may be eaten together as they require an acid or neutral medium for their digestion. But starches and proteins, fats and proteins and starches and acid fruits should not be eaten together as a general rule.

The food combining chart given in the appendix represents diagrammatically food combining rules in an easy-to-follow method. Accompanying this chart is the list of foods in their correct classification. An important point which the elderly should remember about meals is that the smaller the number of courses they consist of, the better it will be. They should approximate to a one-course meal as much as possible. Simple meals in every way are more conducive to health, than more elaborate ones, no matter how well they may be combined.

Daily Menu

Taking the main factors in view, namely supply of all essential nutrients in the diet and balancing the body chemistry and other special requirement of foods, the daily menu of health and vitalising diet for the elderly should be on the following lines:

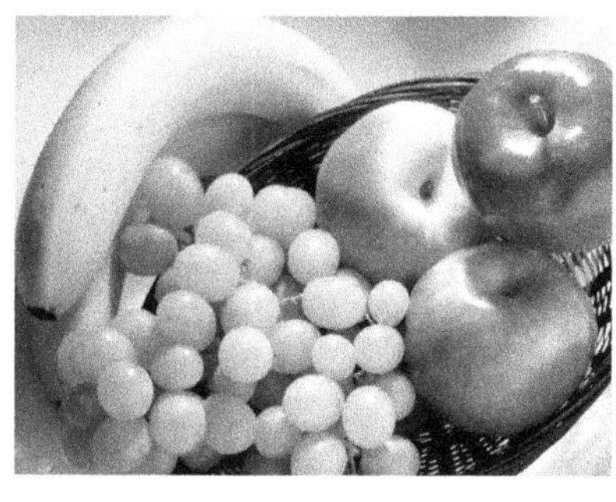

1. Upon arising: A glass of lukewarm water with half freshly-squeezed lime and a teaspoon of honey, or 25 black raisins soaked overnight in water along with water in which they are soaked and water kept overnight in copper vessel, or a glass of freshly-squeezed juice of any available seasonal fruits like apple, pineapple, lemon, orange and grapes.

2. Breakfast: Fresh fruits such as apple, grapes, pear, peaches, pineapple, papaya, a glass of milk sweetened with honey and a few almonds or seeds like sunflower and pumpkin seeds.

3. Lunch: A bowl of freshly-prepared steamed vegetables such as carrot, cabbage, cauliflower, bottle gourd, pumpkin, beans, two or three whole wheat chapatis or cooked brown rice and a glass of buttermilk.

4. Mid-afternoon: A glass of vegetable or fruit juice or coconut water.

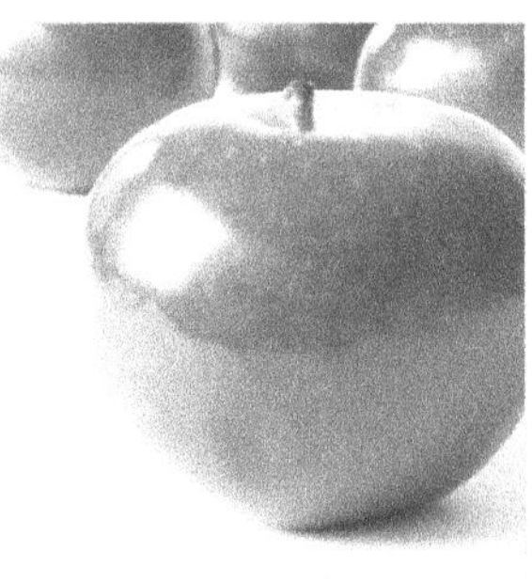

5. Dinner: A bowl of fresh green vegetable salad. Use all available vegetables such as lettuce, carrot, cabbage, cucumber, tomato, radish, red beet onion and sprouts such as alfalfa and mung beans with lemon juice dressing. This may be followed by a hot course such as vegetable soup and a slice of whole meal bread or a small quantity of lightly-cooked vegetables and a whole wheat chapati.

6. Bedtime snack: A glass of milk or one apple.

CHAPTER 3

Vitamins and Minerals Can Slow Down Ageing

It is now recognised that years of faulty nutrition speeds up the process of ageing. Deficiencies of vitamins and minerals can have detrimental effects on the health of the elderly. Recent studies indicate that certain vitamins possess anti-oxidant properties and prevent oxidation process. These vitamins are A, E, C and B-carotene. They can by virtue of these properties delay the ageing process. They also prevent degeneration in blood vessels, heart joints and eye lens.

Vitamins

Among vitamins, the most important are vitamins A, B, C, D and E.

Vitamin A is essential for growth and vitality. It builds up resistance to respiratory and other infections and works mainly on the eyes, lungs, stomach and intestines. It prevents eye diseases and plays a vital role in nourishing the skin and hair.

There are a large variety of vitamins in the B group, the more important being B1 or thiamine, B2 or riboflavin, B3 or niacin or nicotinic acid, B6 or pyridoxine, B9 or folic acid, B12 and B5 or pantothenic acid. Known as anti-beriberi and anti-ageing vitamin,

vitamin B1 plays an important role in the normal functioning of the nervous system, the regulation of carbohydrates and good digestion.

Vitamin B2 is essential for growth and general health and also for healthy eyes, skin, nails and hair. Vitamin B3 is vital for proper circulation, the healthy functioning of the nervous system and for proper protein and carbohydrate metabolism.

Vitamin B6 helps in the absorption of fats and proteins, prevents nervous and skin disorders and protects against degenerative diseases. Vitamin B9, along with vitamin B12, is necessary for the formation of red blood cells. Vitamin B5 stimulates the adrenal glands and increases the production of cortisone and adrenal hormones. Vitamin B12 is essential for the proper functioning of the central nervous system, the production and regeneration of red blood cells and proper utilisation of fat for body building.

Vitamin C is indispensable for normal growth and the maintenance of practically all the body tissues, especially those of the joints, bones, teeth and gums. It protects against infections and acts as a general antibiotic. Vitamin D is necessary for proper bones and teeth formation and for the healthy functioning of the thyroid gland. Vitamin E is must for normal reproductory functions, fertility and physical vigour. It prevents unsaturated fatty acids, sex hormones and fat solvable vitamins from being destroyed in the body by oxygen.

Vitamin C and calcium matter more in old age. Elderly persons who have been deficient in these two nutrients for a long time, will have bones that break easily in a minor fall or injury. Brittle bones are thus not so much due to advancing years as to a serious lack of Vitamin C and calcium. Deficiency of Vitamin C can also lead to weakening of tissues, resulting in rapid ageing. This vitamin also helps to deal effectively with the invading bacteria and viruses that cause infections.

Other diseases which can result from Vitamin C deficiency are pyorrhoea and scurvy. In pyorrhoea, the gums are inflammed and spongy and bleed readily. The bone of the teeth is injured, forming areas of infection. Scurvy, which is quite common in the elderly, can lead to wrinkling, loss of skin elasticity, loss of teeth and brittle bones. A lack of Vitamin C slows down the normal healing processes of the body. The tissue formed to heal wounds, known as scar tissue, requires Vitamin C for its strength.

Research has shown that the body makes heavy demands upon its reserves of Vitamin C during colds, influenza, sinus and catarrhal infections, throat trouble, rheumatic ailments and lung infections. Tests have revealed that patients with these diseases have an extremely low reserve of Vitamin C. Older people suffering from these conditions should, therefore, increase their intake of Vitamin C very considerably. In large daily doses upto 2000 mg. Vitamin C has proved effective in such allergic complaints as hay fever, eczema, asthma and hives. When large doses of Vitamin C are used, calcium should also be taken with it.

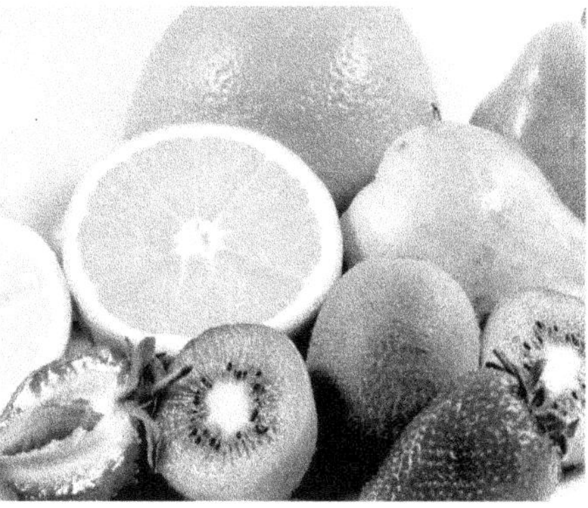

It is considered that as one gets older, the normal Vitamin C intake should be increased. Elderly people bruise easily which is indicative of capillary weakness. Moreover, they often suffer from a lack of hydrochloric acid, which can cause destruction of Vitamin C in the intestines. Any deficiency of hydrochloric acid can be overcome by intake of Vitamin A and the B complex vitamins, as they stimulate the secretion of hydrochloric acid. This in turn will help absorption of Vitamin C effectively.

Another vitamin which is of great value to older persons is Vitamin E. Shortage of this vitamin can prove very harmful in old age. Vitamin E is an essential substance found in every tissue of the body. It protects the cells of the body against incipient destructive oxidation in the wrong places. It dilates the capillaries and enables blood to flow freely into damaged anaemic muscle tissue. It decreases the oxygen requirements of muscle tissue by approximately 50 per cent and diminishes pain and breathlessness. This vitamin dissolves blood clots and prevents their formation. It prevents the formation of excessive scar tissue, and in some instances even melts away unwanted scar tissue.

Vitamin E helps prevent atherosclerosis, strokes and high blood pressure and reduces the risk of heart attacks. Studies have shown that Vitamin E along with selenium can effectively block cancer. Those who have low selenium and Vitamin E in the blood are more prone to develop cancer.

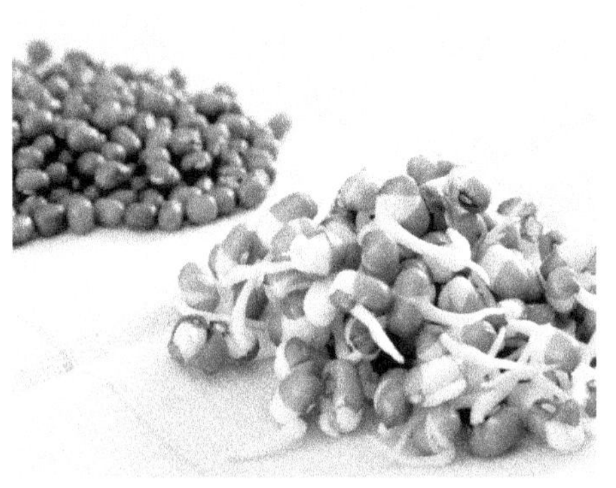

Researchers believe that Vitamin E may be a key factor in slowing the process of ageing. Thus taking sufficient amounts of Vitamin E may enable a person of 60 years to look, feel, act and be more like a person of 50 years. Foods rich in Vitamin E are all whole, raw or sprouted seeds, nuts, whole grain cereals, eggs and green leafy vegetables. These foods retard the ageing process. Vitamin E is now being extensively used by the medical profession in treating a variety of diseases, including male infertility, muscular dystrophy, menopausal disorders and coronary heart diseases.

The Washington-based Alliance for Ageing Research, after 20 years of research, had suggested an upward revision in the recommended daily allowance (RDA) of three anti-oxidant vitamins, the B-carotene (from which the body synthesises Vitamin A), Vitamin C and Vitamin E. All these three vitamins can normally be obtained from fruits and vegetables.

According to the new RDAs, adults should take 250-1000mg. of Vitamin C, 100-400 IU of Vitamin E and 10-30 mg of Beta-carotene every day, to prevent chronic age-related diseases. These allowances are higher by four to 16 times than the current RDAs. These recommendations are aimed at fighting free radicals, the small highly-charged particles, with strong oxidizing power, which contribute to conditions ranging from cancer to atherosclerosis, heart attacks and strokes. The three antioxidant vitamins help to reduce these free radicals and protect other vitamins and minerals from getting destroyed by oxidation.

Minerals

Minerals are vital to health. They are essential for regulating and building the trillions of living cells which make up the body. The more important mineral elements needed by the body are calcium, phosphorous, iron, sulphur, magnesium, sodium, potassium chlorine and iodine.

Calcium, known as the 'wonder mineral', performs many important functions. Without calcium, the contractions of the heart would be faulty, the muscles would not contract properly to make the limbs move and blood would not clot. Calcium stimulates enzymes in the digestive process and coordinates the functions of all other minerals in the body. Phosphorous combines with calcium to create the calcium phosphorus balance necessary for the growth of bones and teeth and in the formation of nerve cells. It is also essential for the assimilation of carbohydrates and fats. It is a stimulant to the nerves and brain. Iron exists chiefly as haemoglobin in the blood. It distributes the oxygen inhaled into the lungs to all the cells. It is the master mineral which creates warmth, vitality and stamina.

The main purpose of sulphur is to dissolve waste minerals. It helps to eject some of the waste and poisons from the system. It helps keep the skin clear of blemishes and makes hair glossy. Magnesium is cool, alkaline, refreshing and sleep-promoting. It assists in the functioning of the nervous system and the composition of nerve and muscle cells. It aids in digestion and in the elimination of waste from the system. Sodium is needed for digestion, blood purification and for the manufacture of gland hormones. It is a necessary constituent of gastric juices and is of utmost importance in neutralising acidity in the body.

Potassium regulates the normal contraction and relaxation of all muscles. It builds up new tissues, flesh, bones and muscles. It also keeps the joints and arteries flexible. Chlorine is necessary for the formation of natural hydrochloric acid in the stomach and also for the manufacture of glandular hormone secretions. It prevents the building of excessive fat and auto-intoxication. Iodine is essential for the formation of thyroxin — the thyroid hormone which regulates much physical and mental activity. It regulates the rate of metabolism, energy production and body weight and helps prevent rough and wrinkled skin.

It has been found that calcium is deficient in the modern diet, and particularly so, in the diet of older people. One of the many purposes of calcium in nutrition is to transport nerve impulses. When it is in short supply, nerves and muscles are tense, leading to irritability and fatigue. A deficiency of this mineral can also cause cramps. Which often appear in old people, usually in the leg muscles or feet.

Insomnia, which is quite common in old age, can be dispelled by the use of calcium, as it relaxes muscles and nerves. Three calcium tablets, taken with a glass of warm milk at bed time, will usually bring sound, refreshing sleep to many older people who do not sleep well. The use of calcium has also been found beneficial in relieving pain. It can be taken in tablet form by older people who are troubled with headache, digestive disorders and arthritis. Other diseases which can be treated by this mineral are menopausal disorders and irritability of nerves and muscles.

The richest sources of calcium are raw milk and unprocessed cheese. Other good food sources are soyabeans, lima beans, string beans, cabbage, cauliflower, dates, molasses, turnip tops, egg yolk, dried figs and lettuce.

Calcium is largely retained in the body by being combined with phosphorus and Vitamin D is necessary before phosphorus can be absorbed efficiently. It follows, therefore that without adequate Vitamin D, phosphorus cannot be utilized; thus a portion of the body's calcium cannot be retained and is excreted from the body.

Vitamin D is important for the proper assimilation of calcium. Older people can readily get this Vitamin by taking a walk in the sunshine. The ultra-violet rays in sunlight cause the oil glands of the skin to secrete a provitamin called ergosterol, which is converted into Vitamin D and absorbed into the body through the skin.

According to Adelle Davis, an eminent nutritionist, the daily menu must include iron. A lack of iron in the diet causes nutritional anaemia, which is characterised by low blood pressure, poor appetite, extreme tiredness, dizziness, forgetfulness and shortness of breath. The most common cause of anaemia is a diet lacking in iron. Another factor responsible for this disease is inadequate hydrochloric acid in the stomach, without which iron cannot be assimilated. With advancing age, the secretion of hydrochloric acid tends to diminish. The vitamins needed to stimulate a flow of hydrochloric acid are Vitamin A, niacinamide and Vitamin B.

Foods rich in iron are liver, wheat germ, whole meal flour, oatmeal unpolished rice, red beets, parsely, carrots, raw onions, apples, bananas and cherries. These foods are more effective in combating simple anaemia than iron pills or tonics, which destroy

Vitamin E in the body. A small quantity of copper, about 2 mgs daily seems to be necessary to enable iron to form haemoglobin. However, many foods rich in iron also contain copper.

Another mineral which is of great importance in old age is iodine. The chief storehouse of iodine in the body is thyroid gland. The essential thyroxine secreted by this gland is made by the circulating iodine. In the body, iodine is converted from the foods rich in this mineral. Thyroxine is a wonder chemical which controls the basic metabolism and oxygen consumption of tissues. It regulates the rate of energy production and body weight and promotes proper growth. It improves mental alacrity and promotes healthy hair, nails, skin and teeth.

Deficiency of iodine can lead to myxedema, which is charecterised by slower rate of metabolism, thickening of the skin, loss of hair, general physical and mental sluggishness and enlarged thyroid gland. Dietary lack may lead to anaemia, fatigue, lethargy, loss of interest in sex, slowed pulse, low blood pressure and a tendency towards obesity. The best dietary sources of iodine are kelp and other seaweeds. Other good sources are turnip greens, garlic, water cress, pineapples, pears, citrus fruits, egg yolks, sea foods and fish liver oils.

CHAPTER 4

Rejuvenative Foods

There are certain foods which prevent mental, physical and sexual senility and prolong youthful vitality and appearance. The usefulness of some of the more important foods noted for such properties are discussed herein in brief.

Almond (Badam)

Known as the king of nuts, almond is a highly nutritious food. It is rich in all essential elements needed by the body.

It is an effective health-building food, both for the body and mind. The chemical substances copper, iron, phosphorus and Vitamin Bl, contained in this nut, exert synergic action and help the formation of new blood cells and haemoglobin. They also play a major role in maintaining the smooth physiological functions of the brain, nerves, bones, heart and liver. Almond is highly beneficial in preserving the vitality of the brain, strengthening the muscles and prolonging life.

Almond is a valuable food remedy for several common ailments, including anaemia, constipation, skin disorders and respiratory diseases. It is very useful in case of loss of sexual energy resulting from nervous debility and brain weakness. Its regular use will strengthen sexual power. The best way to use almonds is to soak them in water and grind them into fine paste, after peeling off the skin.

Amaranth (Chaulai-ka-saag)

The regular use of amaranth, a popular green leafy vegetable, prevents the deficiency of Vitamins A, Bl, B2 and C, calcium, iron and potassium. It protects against several disorders such as defective vision, respiratory infections, recurrent colds, retarded growth and functional sterility.

This vegetable is useful in preventing premature ageing. It prevents disturbance of calcium and iron metabolism. Calcium molecules begin to get deposited in the bone tissues as one grows old. This haphazard calcium distribution is influenced by the improper molecular movements of iron in the tissues. If this molecular disturbance of calcium and iron is prevented by regular supply of food calcium and iron, as in amaranth and the health is maintained from the early age, the process of ageing can be prevented.

Apple (Seb)

The apple is invaluable in the maintenance of good health and in the prevention and treatment of many ailments. This fruit is a highly nutritive food and it contains minerals and vitamins in abundance. It has been found beneficial in the treatment of anaemia, constipation, diarrhoea, dysentery, stomach disorders, headache, heart disease, high blood pressure, rheumatic afflictions, eye and dental disorders.

The various chemicals present in the apple such as Vitamin Bl, phosphorus and potassium help the synthesis of glutamic acid. This chemical substance controls the wear and tear of nerve cells. Eating an apple with honey and milk is very valuable in the nervous disorders like extreme tiredness, lack of concentration, lack of memory, mental irritability and mental depression. It acts as a very effective nerve tonic and recharges the nerves with new energy and life.

The apple is the best fruit to tone up a weak and rundown

condition of the human system. It removes all deficiencies of vital organs and makes the body stout and strong. It tones up the body and the brain as it contains more phosphorus and iron than any other fruit or vegetable. Its regular consumption with milk promotes health and youthfulness and helps build healthy and bright skin. It has a calming and relaxing effect.

Banana (Kela)

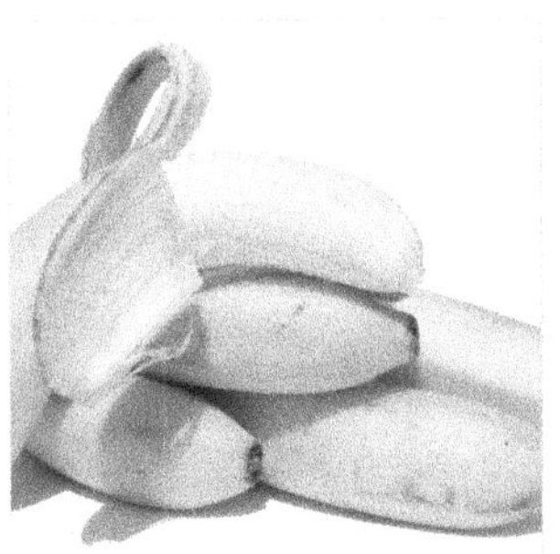

The banana is of great nutritional value. It has a rare combination of energy value, tissue-building elements, protein, vitamins and minerals. It is a good source of calories being richer in solids and lower in water content than any other fresh fruit. A large banana supplies more than 100 calories. It contains a large amount of easily assimilable sugar, making it a good source of quick energy and an excellent means of recovery from fatigue. The use of banana has been found beneficial in the treatment of several disorders, such as intestinal disorders constipation, diarrhoea, dysentery, arthritis, gout, anaemia, allergies, kidney stones, tuberculosis and urinary disorders. Folk physicians of India and ancient Persia regarded this golden fruit as nature's secret of perpetual youth. To this day, banana is known for promoting healthy digestion and helping to create a feeling of youthfulness. It helps promote the retention of calcium, phosphorus and nitrogen which then work to build sound and regenerated tissues. This fruit also contains invert sugar, which is an aid to youthful metabolism.

Cabbage (Pattagobhi)

The cabbage is one of the most highly rated leafy vegetables and a marvellous food item. It is excellent as a muscle builder and cleanser. The most valuable properties of this vegetable are high sulphur and chlorine content and the relatively large percent of iodine. The combination of the sulphur and chlorine causes a cleansing of the mucus membranes of the stomach and intestinal tract, but this only applies when cabbage or its juice is taken in its raw state without the addition of salt. The use of this vegetable has been found valuable in constipation, stomach ulcers, obesity and skin disorders.

This vegetable contains several elements and factors which enhance the immunity of the human body and arrest its premature ageing. Some of these elements help prevent the formation of patches on the walls of blood vessels and stones in the gall bladder. It has been found that a combination of Vitamin P and C in cabbage gives strength to the blood vessels.

Curd (Dahi)

Curd or yoghurt, a lactic fermentation of milk, is a highly versatile and health-promoting food. It is one of the most valuable therapeutic foods. The bacteria, which converts milk into curd, inhibit the growth of hostile or illness-causing bacteria inside the intestinal tract. They also promote beneficial bacteria needed for digestion. These friendly bacteria facilitate the absorption of minerals and aid in synthesis of vitamins of B group. The use of curd has been found valuable in gastrointestinal disorders, insomnia, hepatitis, jaundice and skin disorders.

Curd has been associated with longevity. Elie Metchnikoff, a noble prize-winning Russian bacteriologist at the Pasteur Institute, believed that premature old age and decay could be prevented by taking sufficient curd in the daily diet. He made an intensive study of the problem of old age in the early 1900s. He came to the conclusion that the body is slowly being poisoned and its resistance weakened by man's normal diet and that this poisoning process could be arrested and the intestinal tract kept healthy by the constant and regular use of yoghurt or some variety of acidophilus milk.

Custard Apple (Sitaphal)

The custard apple is one of the most delicious of tropical fruits. It is cool and refreshing to the heart and contains all the body-building elements. It is known for its excellent medicinal properties. This fruit has been found specially valuable in tuberculosis.

The custard apple is said to contain the qualities of the rejuvenating drugs. It increases and maintains blood, sharpens memory, builds up radiant health and prolongs life. As this fruit is rich in fat and protein, it enhances muscular strength and tones up the heart. It has been found to be very useful for the brain and the nervous system. The pulp of the fruit with honey or jaggery can be used as a nutritive tonic by old persons.

Fenugreek (Methi)

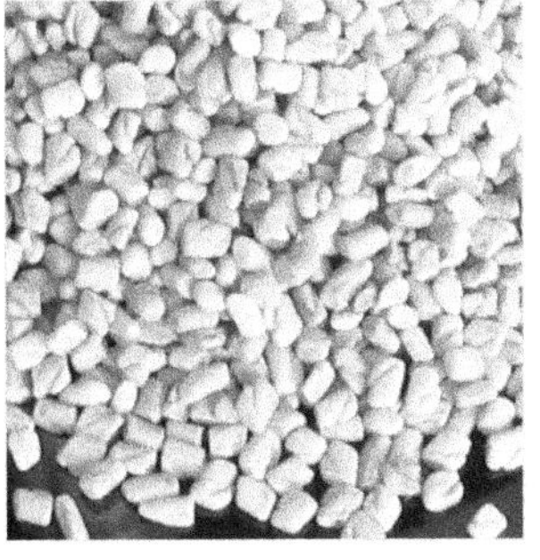

Fenugreek, a well known leafy vegetable, has excellent medicinal properties. Its regular use will help keep the body clean and healthy. The leaves are aromatic, cooling and laxative. They help in blood formation and prevent anaemia. They are considered valuable in indigestion, flatulence and sluggish liver. Steaming is considered the best method of cooking leaves so as to preserve the vitamins contained in them.

The seeds of fenugreek contain an aromatic oil similar in composition to cod-liver oil. This oil accounts for the plant's ancient reputation as a sex rejuvenator. It helps increase sperm count in semen. The seeds also prevent pellagra and nervous disorders. They have been found helpful in controlling diabetes. A tea prepared from fenugreek seeds helps reduce fever, cleanses stomach, bowels, kidneys and respiratory tract of excess mucus.

This tea is prepared by steeping one teaspoon of the seeds in one cup of boiling water. The seeds can also be taken in the form of sprouts or powdered and added to foods and juices.

Garlic (Lahasoon)

The garlic, an important condiment crop, has been held in high esteem for its health-building qualities for centuries all over the world. According to Babhet, an eminent ayurvedic authority, garlic is good for the heart, a food for the hair, a stimulant to appetite and a strengthening food. It is an excellent carminative and nerve tonic. Its marvellous therapeutic value arises from the volatile oil contained in it.

Scientific researchers have found that the garlic is valuable in preventing tuberculosis, pneumonia, diphtheria and typhus and is useful in all respiratory infections, especially in dry hacking coughs, colds, asthma and bronchitis. It relieves dyspepsia, colic and flatulence. It kills round worms and thread worms. It is also good remedy for certain cases of dysentery and diarrhoea. It is also a counter-irritant and rubefacient and can be used with advantage in compress form for pleurisy and tuberculosis of the larynx.

The regular use of garlic, even when one is healthy, imparts strength, increases longevity and keeps one fit to work in old age. Garlic is a natural and harmless aphrodisiac. It is a tonic for loss of sexual power from any cause and for sexual debility and impotency from overindulgence in sex and nervous exhaustion from dissipating habit. It is said to be especially useful to old men of high nervous tension and falling sexual power.

Honey (Shahad)

Honey possesses unique nutritional and medicinal properties. Latest research indicates that the pollen in honey contains all 22 amino acids, 28 minerals, 11 enzymes, 14 fatty acids and 11 carbohydrates. The use of honey has been found valuable in several ailments, including anaemia, pulmonary diseases, irritating cough, insomnia, oral problems, eye afflictions and stomach disorders.

Honey is one of the finest sources of heat and energy, and therefore, very valuable in old age. Energy is generated mainly by the carbohydrate foods and honey is the most easily digested form of carbohydrate. It enters directly into the blood stream because of its dextrine content and this provides instantaneous energy. It is a boon to those with weak digestion. All organs in the body respond favourably when honey is eaten. Famous Roman physician Galen has described honey as an all-purpose medicine for all types of diseases.

Indian Gooseberry (Amla)

Indian gooseberry is a wonderful fruit. It is probably the richest known natural source of Vitamin C which is readily assimilated by the human system. It contributes greatly toward health and longevity. A tablespoon each of fresh gooseberry juice and honey mixed together forms a very valuable medicine for the treatment of several ailments, such as respiratory disorders, diabetes, heart disease, eye disorders, rheumatism, scurvy, diarrhoea and dysentery. Its regular use every morning will promote vigour in the body within a few days.

Indian gooseberry has revitalising effects. It contains an element which is very valuable in preventing ageing and in maintaining strength in old age. It improves body resistance and protects against infection. It strengthens the heart, hair and different glands in the body. It is said that the great ancient sage Muni Chyawan rejuventated himself in his late 70s and regained his virility by the use of amla.

Lettuce (Salad-ka-patta)

Regarded as the king of salad plants, lettuce is a live food with its rich vitamin content, especially the antiscorbutic Vitamin C. It is bulky, low in food value, but high in health value. It is rich in mineral salts with the alkaline elements greatly predominating. So, it helps to keep the blood clean, the mind alert and the body in good health.

Lettuce contains several health-building qualities and thus is very valuable in old age. It has many essential values to the human body. It is very good for brain, nervous system and lungs. The raw juice of lettuce is cool and refreshing. The high content of magnesium in the juice has exceptional power to vitalise the muscular tissues, the nerves and the brain.

Milk (Doodh)

Milk, one of the most common articles of food, occupies a unique position in the maintenance of health and healing of diseases. It is regarded as a complete food. It contains protein, fat, carbohydrates, all the known vitamins, various minerals and all the food ingredients considered essential for sustaining life and maintaining health. The protein of milk is of the highest biological value and it contains all the amino acids essential for body building and repair of body cells. The use of milk has been found especially valuable in fevers, genito-urinary disorders, jaundice, weak teeth, thinness and eye disorders.

According to Charaka, the great author of the Indian system of medicine, milk increases strength, improves memory, removes exhaustion, maintains strength and promotes long life. Experiments conducted in modern times have amply corroborated this opinion of Charaka.

Onion (Piyaz)

Onion, a pungent edible belonging to the same family as garlic, has been described as the dynamite of natural foods. It has been used for centuries for the treatment of a wide range of diseases

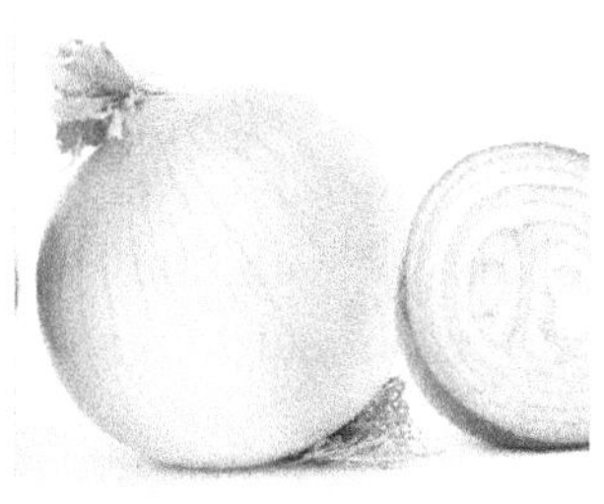

such as cold, cough, bronchitis, influenza, tuberculosis, anaemia, bleeding piles, dropsy, tooth and ear disorders. It stimulates the circulation of blood in mucous membranes and is regarded as a potent germ killer. Chewing an onion for five minutes destroys all harmful bacteria in the lining of the mouth.

Onion is being used as therapeutic agent for treating high blood pressure and other problems of the circulatory system. This vegetable boiled or fried can help reduce the possibility of heart attacks by raising the blood's capacity to dissolve or prevent deadly internal clots.

Onion is one of the most important of aphrodisiac foods and is second only to garlic in this respect. It increases libido and strengthens the reproductory organs. The white variety of onion should be peeled off, crushed and fried in pure butter. This mixture acts as an excellent aphrodisiac tonic if taken regularly with a spoon of honey on an empty stomach.

Research has shown that onion emits a peculiar type of ultraviolet radiation called M-rays. It appears to stimulate cell activity and produce a rejuvenating effect in the system.

Raisins (Munaqqa)

Raisins are dried grapes. They are esteemed for their high food value, which arise chiefly from their sugar content. They contain eight times more sugar than grapes. The sugar contained in them is of superior quality. A major portion of this sugar is formed by glucose and fruit sugar, which produce quick heat and energy in the body. Raisins are thus an excellent food in all cases of debility. Their use has been found specially valuable in acidosis, constipation, anaemia, thinness and febrile cases.

Black raisins are used for restoration of sexual vigour. They should be boiled with milk, after washing them thoroughly in tepid water. This will make them puffy and sweet. Eating of these raisins should be followed by consumption of milk. Starting with 30 gms of raisins with 200 ml. of milk, three times daily, the quantity of raisins should be gradually increased to 50 gms each time.

Soyabean (Bhatma)

The soyabean is high in food value. It is a very valuable source of protein, vitamins, minerals and other food ingredients. Its protein is of great biological value. It is 'complete' as it contains all the essential amino acids or building blocks of protein in the proportions that make them most available for human needs. It is the best of all vegetable proteins and ranks in this respect with protein of milk, egg and meat. But soyabean contains by far more protein than these articles. While most proteins are acid in their ash, soyabean is rich in alkaline-bearing salts and hence regarded as a corrective diet.

Soyabean, especially in the form of milk, is very valuable in old age. It is an excellent nerve tonic. It is useful in nervous disorders like mental irritability, nervous tension, insomnia, forgetfulness and neuritis. It tones up the nervous system due to its rich concentration of lecithin, Vitamin Bl, phosphorus and glutamic acid. For better results, a cupful of soyabean milk should be mixed with a teaspoonful of honey and taken every night.

Sunflower (Suryamukhi) Seeds

Sunflower seeds, the most familiar of all edible seeds, are the tightly packed core of the glorious sunflowers. They are well above average in protein, phosphorus and iron concentration and very rich source of B-complex vitamins. They are almost 50 per cent fat which makes them a highly satisfying food that prevents the let-down feeling of fatigue and weariness that comes with age.

Sunflower seeds are highly beneficial in old age. They contain substantial quantity of linoleic acid which is the fat helpful in reducing cholesterol deposits on the walls of arteries. They help to protect the health of nerves and brain as well as skin and digestive tract. Their use has been found valuable in anaemia and respiratory diseases like bronchitis, tonsillitis, influenza and cough. The seeds can be sprinkled over cereals, salads, yoghurt and soups or mixed with vegetables.

Wheat (Gehun)

Wheat, the most widely used cereal for making bread, is a good source of energy. Every part of the wheat grain supplies elements needed by the human body. Starch and gluten in wheat provide heat and energy; the inner bran coats, phosphates and other mineral salts; the outer bran, the much-needed roughage; the germ, Vitamins B and E; and its protein helps build and repair muscular tissue. The whole wheat, which includes bran and wheat germ, thus provides protection against diseases such as constipation, ischaemic heart disease, diverticular disease of the colon and thus prolongs life.

Wheat grass, which is grown by spreading the soaked wheat grains in earth-filled earthen pots, is a wonder plant. It is an extremely rich source of chlorophyll, which can be utilised as a body cleanser, rebuilder and neutraliser of toxins. It also contains several minerals. Wheat juice furnishes the body with vital nourishment, providing extra energy to the body. The regular drinking of this juice removes toxins from the body, maintains good health and prolongs life. It is also valuable in the prevention and treatment of several skin diseases, digestive system maladies and circulatory disorders.

CHAPTER 5

Harmful Foods that Hasten Ageing

There is a growing tendency in modern times to make the articles of diet as artificial and pleasing to the eye as possible and tasty to the tongue, without any regard to their ultimate effect on health. This has led to the refining and demineralising of cereals and sugar and addition of salt to various foodstuffs to make them tasty and delicious. Fortunately, there is realisation now among the enlightened people that the artificial and concentrated dietary, to a large extent, is responsible for the vast array of present-day diseases.

Foods such as bread, cereals and sugar are very acid-forming, if eaten in the refined state as white bread, white sugar and polished rice. But these foods are far less acid-forming in character if eaten in the natural state as natural brown sugar, as whole meal bread and as natural brown rice. The excessive use of salt also leads to the formation of acids in the body.

Of the various artificial foodstuffs being used today for their delicious taste, white flour, sugar and salt, known as three white products, have been found especially harmful. Similarly, excessive consumption of tea and coffee is very injurious to health and can lead to weakening of the system. The harmful effects of all these foods are discussed in this chapter.

White Flour

Wheat is the most common cereal used throughout the world for making bread. It is good source of energy. With its essential coating of bran, vitamins and minerals, it is an excellent health-building food.

The wheat grain is a seed which consists of three main parts, namely, the various outer coverings, endosperm and the germ or embryo. The outer coverings contain much indigestible fibre. Beneath them is the aluerone layer which is rich in protein. Inside is the endosperm which consists of an inner and outer portion. The germ or embryo which consists of the shoot and root. It is attached to the grain by a special structure, the scutellum.

The germ of the wheat is relatively rich in protein, fat and several of the B Vitamins. So is the scutellum which contains 50 times more thiamine than the whole grain. The outer layers of the endosperm and the aleurone layer contains a higher concentration of protein, vitamins and phytic acid than the inner endosperm. The inner endosperm contains most of the starch and protein in the grain.

Wheat is usually ground into flour before use as food. In ancient times, wheat grains were crushed between two large stones. This method preserved all parts of the Kernel and the product was called "whole wheat." If it is finely ground, it becomes whole wheat four. The value of stone grinding is that the grain is ground slowly and it remains unheated, and a whole food. In modern times, steel roller mills have superseded stone grinding. These mills grind wheat a hundred times faster, but they impoverish the flour by removing the precious wheat germ, resulting in colossal loss in vitamins and minerals in the refining process. The following tables show the food values of various types of wheat (per cent per 100 gms).

Type of Wheat	Moisture gm.	Protein gm.	Fat gm.	Minerals gm.	Fibre gm.	Carbohydrates gm.	Energy gm.
Wheat (Whole)	12.8	11.8	1.5	1.5	1.2	71.2	346
Wheat Flour (Whole)	12.2	12.1	1.7	2.7	1.9	69.4	341
Wheat Flour (Refined)	13.3	11.0	0.9	0.6	0.3	73.9	348
Wheat Germ	5.2	29.2	7.4	3.5	1.4	53.5	397

Type of Wheat	Carotene Mcg.	Thiamine Mg.	Riboflavin Mg.	Niacin Mg.	Calcium Mg.	Phosphorus Mg.	Iron Mg.
Wheat (Whole)	64	0.45	0.17	5.5	41	306	4.9
Wheat Flour (Whole)	29	0.49	0.29	4.3	48	355	11.5
Wheat Flour (Refined)	25	0.12	0.07	2.4	23	121	2.5

In the refining of whole wheat, the precious wheat germ is removed. By doing so, we remove the very life of the grain of wheat, because locked in the wheat germ is an oil which is man's greatest food. The wheat germ also contains all-important Vitamin E, known as the anti-sterility factor or sex vitamin. A lack of this vitamin can also lead to heart disease. The colossal loss of vitamins and minerals in the refined wheat flour has lead to widespread prevalence of constipation and other digestive disturbances and nutritional disorders.

White Sugar

Sugar is the most common sweet carbohydrate used all over the world. There are many varieties of sugar, but only a few are included, to any considerable extent, in our diet. These are sucrose or cane sugar, dextrose or grape sugar, levulose or fruit sugar and lactose or milk sugar. Natural sugar contained in fruits is called fructose.

Cane sugar, also called the white sugar, is produced in enormous quantities. It is derived commercially from the sugar cane and beet root. When it is eaten, it is slowly converted into levulose and dextrose, for it cannot be utilised by the body in its native form. It must first undergo a digestive process as does starch. But, unlike starch, the digestion of cane sugar does not begin in the mouth, but is delayed until the sugar reaches the intestine.

There has been enormous increase in the consumption of sugar all over the world. Commensurate with the sharp rise of sugar consumption, there has been an alarming increase in the incidence of several diseases. There is mounting evidence from many medical sources that white sugar is extremely injurious to health. The heat and chemical process employed in the sugar refinery kills the vitamins and separates the mineral elements, protein and other substance from the sap, leaving nothing but pure sugar crystals, robbed of mineral elements and the life-sustaining vitamins.

White sugar has many great disadvantages. It is irritating and it is difficult to digest. It is called the vitamin thief. Its high intake can rob the body of its vitamins made available to it by consumption of other foods. Excessive use of white sugar leads to gastric catarrh and hyperacidity. It is also associated with obesity, dental caries, diabetes and coronary heart disease.

The white sugar supplies only calories without any nutritive value. It contains as many as 390 calories per 100 gms. It has been estimated that 90 per cent of overweight persons consume much more sugar than required. Eating sugar adds to calories. These are stored in the form of fat.

Another problem with sweet foods is that they can easily be overeaten because of their delicious taste. Cakes, pastries, biscuits and chocolates are some of the items that have a high sugar content and therefore have many calories. For instance, half a small bar of chocolate provides same amount of calories as five apples, but it does not contain the nutrients and fibre that the fruit provides. Thus, if two apples are eaten, it gives a sense of satisfaction due to its fibre content and less calories are ingested. On the other hand, while eating chocolates or sweets, more and more can be eaten without a sense of fullness and therefore, more calories are ingested, leading to obesity.

The most harmful effects of sugar is on the teeth. It dissolves quickly in saliva and finds its way into the bacterial layer on the teeth, known as plaque. It feeds on sugar and converts into acid. This acid eats away the enamel and causes cavities. This acid is produced within seconds of the sugar entering the mouth and attacks the tooth enamel as long as the sugar remains in contact with the teeth. For this reason, both the amount of sugar eaten and its frequency during the day, are important. Sugary foods like biscuits, cakes, fruits and drinks, taken often between the meals, therefore, cause tooth decay. Sticky foods such as toffee and dry fruits that cling to the teeth, are particularly harmful.

Dr. D. T. Quigley, MD, an eminent medical authority, says: "Sugar is a concentrated carbohydrate, containing no vitamin or mineral of any kind. Every ounce of sugar that is taken reduces the ability to resist infection, as it furnishes only calories and none of the elements which protect against infection."

Natural sugars such as brown sugar, unsulphured dark molasses and honey, are preferable to refined white sugar, because they possess some vitamins and minerals. Raw honey also contains enzymes.

White Salt

Man's need for sodium chloride, the chemical name for the common salt, has been a subject of dispute since the beginning of medical practice. The first known salt mines have been found in the Austrian Tyrol and date from the late Bronze Age, about 1,000 B.C. It is not known accurately when man first began to use salt. However, salt was available in the early civilisation and Homer called it 'divine.'

Sodium chloride is a chemical compound found in the sea soil and it also occurs naturally in foods. It is made up of two chemicals, namely, sodium, an element which never occurs in free form in nature, 40 per cent and chloride 60 per cent.

Sodium chloride is a major factor in maintaining acid-base equilibrium of the body. It is also needed for the working of various nerves and muscles of the body and helps in transmitting nerve impulses. It can help prevent catarrh. It promotes a clear brain, resulting in a better disposition and less mental fag. Because of its influence on calcium, sodium can also help dissolve any stones forming within the body, in the kidneys, urinary bladder and gallbladder. It is also essential for the production of hydrochloric acid in the stomach.

Thus, a certain amount of salt in the system is essential for life, but it is required in very small amounts, ranging from 10 to 15 gms daily, depending on the climate and occupation of the person. Many people, however, use too much salt. This puts an extra burden on the kidneys and may cause high blood pressure.

Too much salt in the body can result in oedema or swelling of the legs and ankles. This is due to incomplete elimination of salt through the kidneys. The blood pressure may rise and may not go down again until the excess sodium has been removed from the body.

Intake of too much salt can attract water, creating an artificial thirst. So a person drinks enormous quantities of water and this leads to obesity in due course. Excessive intake of salt can also lead to stomach ulcer, stomach cancer, hardening of arteries and heart disease.

The adverse effects of excessive use of sodium chloride can be rectified by avoiding the use of common salt. Even foods rich in salt such as salted nuts, biscuits, meat, fish, chicken, egg, cheese, dried fruits, spinach, carrot and radish should be avoided. However, low-sodium foods like cereals, sugar, honey, fresh fruits, brinjals, cabbage, cauliflower, tomatoes, potatoes, onions, peas and pumpkin can be used.

It will also be advisable to omit salt altogether in case of all chronic diseases like high blood pressure, arthritis and allergies. In case total avoidance is not possible, it may be added in a very small quantity after cooking. This will prevent it from getting into every particle of the food, which will happen if salt is added before cooking. Salt added after cooking will be just superficial and only to satisfy the taste.

Tea and Coffee

Of all the beverages, tea and coffee are the most widely consumed drinks by people all over the world. These beverages are taken mainly as hot drinks for their stimulating effect. They help to get over a tired feeling and one feels refreshed after drinking. This reputation leads to tea and coffee drinking habits which later become deep-rooted.

The rapid spread of tea and coffee is a striking example of the manner in which commercial forces cultivate poison habits in man for profit. It is believed that almost a billion cups of tea are consumed daily all over the world. In India, even slogans like *Roz Chai Piyo, Bahut Din Jiyo* were invented by the vested interests to mislead common people to believe that tea gives strength and vitality.

Tea

Tea is prepared from the leaves of an evergreen shrub belonging to Camellia family. The plant is native to South East Asia. In ancient times, the leaves were probably eaten or boiled into a beverage. The earliest record of its cultivation comes from China in the fourth century A.D. By the eighth century, it was quite popular in China and established in Japan. Over the next 600 years or so, the method of infusing tea in water slowly evolved.

Tea was introduced into Europe in the 17th century and was at first a great luxury. After the discovery that tea could be grown easily on large estates in Sri Lanka and India, enormous quantities were imported into Great Britain, where for nearly a century and a half it has been a cheap and popular beverage. However, it was not a popular drink in India even as late as 1940.

The Second World War brought about a sharp rise in the prices of commodities all over the world, including India, owing to scarcity of food. As a result, the common people could not afford milk in adequate quantities due to six-fold increases in its price. Deprived of this nutritious food, they turned to tea as a substitute.

To ascertain the effect of tea on health, it is essential to know the chemical composition of tea leaves. On an average, they contain moisture (5 to 8 per cent), aromatic oils (0.5 per cent), caffeine (2.5 to 5 per cent), nitrogen (4.75 to 5.5 per cent), soluble matter (38 to 45 per cent), tannin (7 to 14 per cent) and minerals (5 to 5.75 per cent).

Of these ingredients, the most important are the alkaloids caffeine, tannin and a small proportion of an aromatic oil. The chief effects of tea are due to these ingredients. It is well known that Indian tea is richer in all these chief ingredients than the Chinese variety.

It is not the composition of leaves alone that affects the health but also the composition of infusion which is prepared by boiling tea with water. It is noted that caffeine comes out more rapidly than tannin and hence the greater the period of infusion, the more is the amount of tannin, while the amount of caffeine will remain almost the same.

It will be seen from the composition of tea leaves that tea cannot be regarded as a food and whatever little nutritional value it has is due to milk and sugar which are added to it.

The use of tea is detrimental to health. Dr. P. C. Roy, father of modern chemistry in India, equated tea with poison. Tea is said to slow down digestion. Its daily intake causes indigestion as it impedes the action of 'ptyalin,' a digestive ferment of saliva which acts on cooked starch. The inhibition of saliva seems to be due to tannin. The effect disappears if milk is added to it, as the protein of milk precipitates the tannin. Tea is also said to delay stomach digestion. It can lead to gas formation, diarrhoea and constipation.

Caffeine has a diuretic effect. Experiments show that caffeine in five cups of tea increases the urine by 400 to 500 per cent. This continued stimulation of kidneys by caffeine may damage them.

The stimulating and restorative effects of tea are due to the action of caffeine on the nervous system. It affects the higher cerebral or psychic centres more than centres located in medulla and spinal cord. This results in heightening of intellectual faculties, relieving a feeling of fatigue and increasing the capacity for physical and mental work.

The respiratory and cardiac centres are also stimulated by caffeine as coronary arteries get dilated resulting in increase in the rate of blood flow. It is also said to increase the blood sugar level. The quickening of respiration lowers the level of carbon dioxide and increases the heat production of the body by 10 to 20 per cent.

It is thus clear that tea, if taken in excess, causes indigestion, over-excitability of the nervous system, irritability, palpitation and sometimes prostration. To minimize the harmful effects of tea, it should be infused by pouring water brought to a boil instantly over the leaves and the tea allowed to draw for about four to five minutes, then the liquid should be poured into another pot. Mint and lemon grass should be added. This will help in stomach disorders like flatulence.

Coffee

Coffee beans are the seeds of coffee trees that are widely cultivated in the tropics. There are a variety of coffee trees. Most of them are 10 to 15 ft. high, with evergreen leaves. Shade trees are necessary to protect them from excessive sun. They bear clusters of white flowers which develop into the beans. There are large plantations in India, Indonesia, Africa and Brazil.

Coffee is a native of Africa, where it has been cultivated for ages on the slopes of Abyssinia facing the Red Sea. The coffee tree crossed the sea and found its way into Arabia in the 15th century. The world derives its famous Mocha coffee from there.

Coffee drinking spread very rapidly in the East but entered Europe more slowly. It was imported into England in about 1652. But it was not until the 18th century that coffee drinking was generally adopted. It is, however, about two centuries, since it became an article of general consumption by the people of Europe. In the United states, about 96 per cent of the families drink coffee daily.

Coffee is even more injurious to health than tea. It is a more stimulating beverage than tea, as it contains greater amount of the active alkaloid principle, caffeine. This alkaloid is habit-forming and can be fatal to both man and animal. Sir Robert Hutchison, an eminent nutritionist, found about 100 mg of caffeine and 200 mg of tannin in a cupful of coffee, made by infusing 60 g in 450 ml of water.

Research studies have shown that coffee drinking has potential health hazards. They have linked it to heart disease, cancer and even birth defects. The most common side-effects of coffee are nervousness, irritability, heart palpitation and insomnia.

Coffee drinking can also cause diarrhoea, headache and heartburn. In some people, coffee acts as a diuretic and they may have enormous increase in urine output. Some people experience a post-stimulation letdown that can make them as tired and lethargic as they were alert and energetic immediately after drinking.

A study on role of coffee in heart disease, done at Stanford University, found that sedentary man between 30 and 55, who drink three cups of coffee or more a day may be at higher risk of developing heart disease than those who drink less coffee. There is some indication that heavy coffee consumption, when accompanied by other diet and lifestyle factors, may increase cholesterol levels.

Coffee should be completely given up by those suffering from peptic ulcers, heartburn and other gastrointestinal disorders such as esophageal reflux, as it promotes gastric-acid secretion. People with hypertension, heart disease and anaemia should also avoid coffee. It inhibits the absorption of iron. Researchers at Yale University found that caffeine produces a more pronounced reaction in people who have panic episodes than in normal healthy people.

There are also several studies that indicate a link between coffee-tea drinking and fibrocystic breast disease, a condition characterised by benign breast lumps. Women with these conditions should therefore refrain from drinking these beverages.

To reduce the adverse effects of coffee on health, it should be made by the filter or percolator. Methods have been devised to remove most of the caffeine from coffee, making it caffeine less coffee. Coffee substitutes are made from roasted cereals. They resemble coffee in the bitter taste and aroma. Cereal coffee varieties are wholesome and are used extensively by healthy-minded people and by those desirous of breaking the coffee habit.

CHAPTER 6

Herbs to Fight Old Age

There are certain herbs which have been reputed to build up health and prolong life. They contain elements which are conducive to longevity. Some of these herbs have been found to contain very powerful anti-oxidants, more powerful than the artificial anti-oxidants added to our food as preservatives. The usefulness of some of the more important herbs considered valuable in increasing the life span are described in brief in this chapter.

Alfalfa

Alfalfa, botanically known as Medico satina, is one of the most nutritionally versatile plants yet discovered. Its seeds, leaves and stems provide valuable properties for human beings and grazing animals alike. The Arabs, who discovered this herb, called it the king of kings of plants and the Father of all foods. The Persians knew it as one of Nature's most healing grasses.

Alfalfa is a valuable source of Vitamins A, B, D, E and G. It also has some Vitamin C and blood clotting Vitamin K. Of special value in alfalfa is the rich quality, quantity and proper balance of calcium, sodium, magnesium, phosphorous, chlorine, potassium and silicon. These elements are all very much needed for the proper functioning of the various organs in the body. This herb is one of the richest chlorophyll foods that builds up both animals and humans into a healthy and vigorous old age.

Alfalfa is an outstanding alkalizing food, which makes it a valuable food remedy for several ailments. It increases the peristalsis of the bowels, improves digestion and ensures better assimilation of food. Alfalfa, in the form of juice, extracted from its leaves, has been found very helpful in most troubles with the arteries and heart disease. This juice is also useful in the respiratory disorders. Alfalfa in the form of seeds, known as king of sprouts, is of immense value in building up an immunity to stomach disorders. A tea made from these seeds is highly beneficial in the treatment of arthritis and high blood pressure.

Brahmi

Brahmi, botanically known as Herpestis Monniera or Bacopa Monniera, is a well-known Indian herb. It is generally found in moist or wet places, such as borders of water channels, wells and irrigated fields in all parts of the country. The herb is a cardiac and nervine tonic and it purifes the blood. It strengthens mental faculties and its use has been found valuable in several diseases, including nervous disorders, loss of memory, stoppage of urine, rheumatism and debility — the conditions which are quite common in old age.

Brahmi is reputed as a herb for longevity. Its regular use increases vitality, strengthens the various organs of the body and helps to fight diseases and old age. It has been mentioned in ancient Indian Medical treatise '*Charak Samitha*' that this herb cures all kinds of diseases and bestows longevity. It is said that a person named Jinchigiyan of China attained the age of 250 years by the regular use of this Indian herb. An eminent British scientist, after extensive study of brahmi, reported that this small herb possesses the miraculous property of curing various diseases, and that if only two leaves of this herb are eaten daily, it adds to the vitality and longevity considerably.

Chebulic Myrobalan (Harad or Haritaki)

Chebulic Myrobalan, botanically known as Terminalia chebula retz, is a miraculous herb and is known as long-life elixir. There is an old Indian proverb which says: "If one bites a piece of haritaki everyday after meals and swallows its juice, he will remain free from all diseases."

Chebulic Myrobalan is a mild, safe, and efficacious laxative. It is useful in correcting disordered processes of nutrition and restores the normal functions of the system. This herb is one of the ingredients of the famous Ayurvedic preparation triphala, which is used in the treatment of enlarged liver stomach disorders and pain in the eyes. The use of this herb has been found beneficial in the treatment of hyperacidity, heart-burn, asthma, constipation, diarrhoea, dysentery and piles. A decoction made from chebulic myrobalan is popular gargle for mouth inflammation. This decoction, used as a wash, relieves eye congestion.

Cowhage (Kaunch or Kavatch)

Cowhage, botanically known as Mukuna Prurita, is a famous creeper, with kidney-bean shaped flowers and seeds. It occurs all over India. The roots of this herb are stimulant and tonic and the seeds are nutritive and nervine tonic. The use of this herb has been found valuable in old age as it imparts vigour and vitality. It is also useful in nervous disorders, dropsy, cholera, delirium and bone fractures.

Cowhage is a highly aphrodisiac herb, found beneficial in sexual debility and weakness. One gram dose of the powdered root should be taken with milk to treat this condition. The seeds of the herb are valuable in spermatorrhoea or thinness of semen. They are ingredients of several commercial preparations which are said to have beneficial effects in the management of various sexual disorders.

Ginseng

Ginseng is a wonder herb, with outstanding medicinal properties. It has been used in China, Korea, Japan, India and Southeast Asia for its vitalizing and restorative powers and as a remedy for several ailments for over 5,000 years.

Li-Shin-Chen, a noted Chinese physician who lived towards the end of the 16th century, hailed ginseng root as an aphrodisiac and prescribed it for a variety of diseases. Medical reporter Paul M. Kourennoff in his exhaustive work Russian Folk Medicine, says, 'what was confirmed by all European doctors practising in the Orient was that the use of ginseng medications has an extraordinary effect upon the metabolism of all takers, and dramatically improved the general tone of their system.'

Modern scientific studies on ginseng have found that the herb emits a mitogenetic ray which is considered an all-natural ultra-violet radiation. Nature has put within ginseng a process of cellular proliferation via this mitogenetic emission. It is said that this all-natural cellular rejuvenation process stimulates the body's own sluggish processes and thereby promotes the youth-building benefit of cellular renewals — the key to healing and regeneration.

Ginseng can be used in various ways. The hard and dry root can be sliced into pieces, steamed for 5 to 10 minutes and chewed. The dry root can be grated and powdered and taken in doses of half a teaspoon, mixed in a cup of boiled water, after flavouring with cinnamon. This powder can also be taken mixed in a fresh fruit juice, after thorough stirring.

Holy Basil (Tulsi)

The holy basil is a well-known sacred plant of the Indians. The leaves and seeds of the plant are medicinal. The leaves are tonic. They sharpen memory, remove catarrhal matter and phlegm from the bronchial tubes, strengthen the stomach and induce copious perspiration. They are specific for many fevers. A decoction of the

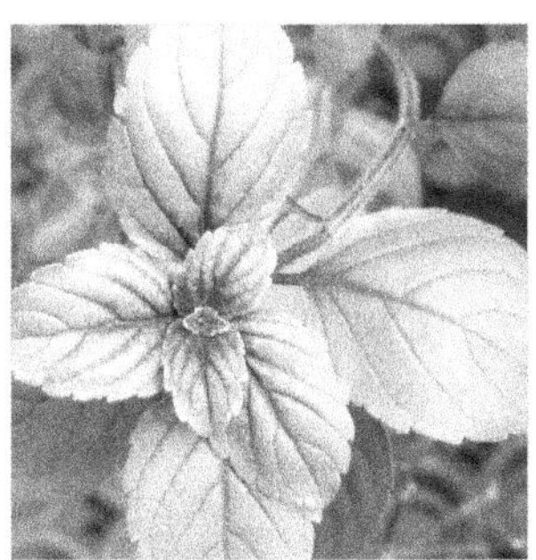

leaves boiled with powdered cardamom in half a litre of water and taken mixed with honey and milk, will bring down the temperature. A decoction of the leaves, mixed with honey and ginger, is an effective remedy for bronchitis, asthma, influenza, cough and cold. The use of basil has been found beneficial in cardiac diseases and in reducing the level of blood cholesterol.

The basil leaves are regarded as adaptogen or anti-stress agent. Recent studies have shown that the leaves protect against stress significantly. It has been suggested that even healthy persons should chew 12 leaves of basil twice daily, morning and evening, for preventing stress. It will also purify the blood and help prevent several common ailments, thereby prolonging life.

Pollen

Pollen refers to the fine powder, usually yellow in colour found inside the blossoms of herbs and flowers. It has been mentioned in texts of Babylon, Egypt, Persia and China that this remarkable plant substance held the magic key to the secret of strength, health and longevity. Today, primitive tribes who live a more natural life, cherish it as a youth sustainer and valuable remedy for many ailments.

In 1945, Nicolai Tsitsin, a Russian biologist, questioned 50 people in Russia who claimed to be over 100 years of age. He made a very interesting discovery that a large number of them were bee keepers and all of them ate waste matter in the bottom of the beehive, a large part of which was almost pure pollen.

Scientists in different countries have carried out experiments with pollen. They agree that hardly a foodstuff exists in either the vegetable or animal kingdom in which so many varied essentials of digestive needs are so completely united as in the case of pollen. Researchers in Switzerland have shown that it contains protein, free amino acids, various forms of sugar, mucilage, fats, minerals, trace elements, large quantities of the Vitamin B complex and also Vitamins A, D, E and C. It also contains uncounted diastase and hormone components and antibiotics, besides other active ingredients not yet known. They conclude that various elements of pollen work together to keep a person more youthful even in old age.

Rosemary (Rusmary)

Rosemary, a sweet-scented herb, has been found valuable in old age. It has long been regarded as the herb for the remembrance. Mystically, it symbolises loyalty, love and immortality. It was once believed to strengthen the heart as well as the memory. The Greeks and Romans prepared a fragrant distilled water from the flowers and inhaled the odour so that "the evils were destroyed from the mind and the memory no longer played tricks."

Rosemary is considered valuable in affections of the head and nerves. It strengthens the sight and memory. It is an antidote to mental fatigue and forgetfulness. A tea made from the herb is considered highly beneficial for tiredness. It is refreshing and a good natural remedy for bringing added mental agility. It is believed that if the crushed leaves of rosemary are inhaled, keeping the eyes closed, the mind will become crystal clear as the vapour penetrates the brain cells. The oil of rosemary can be taken internally in doses of a few drops as a stimulant. A five per cent tincture is used as circulatory and cardiac stimulant.

Sage (Salvia or sefakuss)

Sage, one of the most important culinary herbs, has always played a great role in the history of botanic medicine. The Chinese adage 'sage for old age' sums up its healthful qualities. It has a reputation to retard old age, restore energy and aid digestion. It has a centuries-old reputation of exerting a beneficial influence on the brain, nerves, eyes and glands. Gerard, the famous herbalist, found sage effective for "quickening the senses and memory, strengthening the sinews and restoring health to those suffering from palsies which cause shaking and trembling of limbs."

Sage has been found useful in failing memory. It acts on the cortex of the brain thereby eliminating mental exhaustion and improving concentration. The herb is also valuable in coping with stress. A tea made from the leaves should be taken in this condition. This tea is prepared by pouring a cup of boiling water over one teaspoon of dried sage leaves. The water should be covered and the leaves infused for several minutes. It should then be strained and sweetened with honey, if desired. In case of fresh sage leaves, a tablespoon of coarsely chopped leaves should be used and tea prepared in the same manner.

CHAPTER 7

Exercise and Yoga Can Retard Ageing Process

Exercise plays an important role in maintaining good health and in preventing the ageing process. According to the Journal of American Geriatrics. "If an inactive 70-year-old were to begin an exercise programme of 'moderate activity', the result would be a gain of 15 years.... If the subject were to achieve the 'athlete' level of conditioning, there would be a potential improvement of 40 years!"

Medical researchers at Harvard and Stanford Universities, who studied the habits and health of 17,000 middle-aged and older men, also reported the first scientific evidence that even modest exercise helps prolong life. Dr. Ralph S.R Paffenbarger, the visiting professor of epidemiology at the Harvard School of Public Health, who is the principal author of the report, said, "We have found a direct relationship between the level of physical activity and the length of life in the college men we have studied. He added, "this is the first good evidence that people who are active and fit have a longer life span than those who are not."

A parallel research report from doctors in Dulles also concluded, after studying the lives and habits of 6,000 men and women, that the physically fit were less likely to develop hypertension. Dr. Steven N. Blair who headed the research group said, "We followed the physical health and habits of these people for an average of four and a half years and the data showed that the lack of physical fitness leads to hypertension."

Systematic physical exercise relaxes and softens contracted muscles, ligaments and other tissues and tones up those which are weakened. It promotes blood circulation, expands the lungs, thereby increasing the intake of oxygen, stimulates the appetite and helps in the elimination of waste and morbid matter through the skin, lungs, kidneys and bowels. It also promotes physical strength and mental vigour and strengthens will power and self control, leading to a harmonious development of the whole system.

Exercise increases calorie output. The body fat can be reduced by regular exercise. It is, therefore, useful for weight reduction in conjunction with restricted food intake. According to a study by Dr. Peter Wood of Stanford University Medical School, the author of 'California Diet and Exercise Programme,' very active people eat about 600 more calories daily than their sedentary counterparts but weigh about 20 per cent less. Up to 15 hours after vigorous exercise, the body continues to burn calorie at a higher rate than it would have without exercise. Moderate physical exercise has been found to be accompanied by less obesity and lower cholesterol levels.

Regular exercise plays an important role in the fight against stress by providing recreation and mental relaxation, besides keeping the body physically and mentally fit. It is nature's best tranquiliser.

The proper distribution of nutrients to all parts of the body is closely linked with the exercising of those parts. If any part of the body is allowed to remain idle, it will become weak and defective. Indeed, the joint action of all parts of the body is vital for circulation and the optimum physical functioning. Exercise, besides being one of the most powerful factors in preventing disabilities of later age, is also an important form of therapy for repairing the damage caused by various ailments. It also reduces the risk for all types of cancer by significantly boosting the body's internal defences against free radicals.

Several systems of exercise have been developed over the years. The most popular among them are Swedish system and yogasanas. Whichever system one chooses to adopt, the exercises should be performed systematically, regularly and under proper guidance. To be really useful, exercise should be taken in such a manner as to bring into action all the muscles of the body in a natural way. Walking is one such exercise. It can help reduce weight, give more energy and tone up flabby muscles. It can help prevent heart disease, alleviate mental depression and ease some of the pain of arthritis as well as reverse some of the physical aspects of ageing. Walking is, however, so gentle in character that one must walk several kilometres in brisk manner to constitute a fair amount of exercise. Other forms of good exercise are swimming, bicycling, horse-riding and playing tennis.

Yoga

Yoga is an ancient system of discipline practised in India. It aims at entire well-being of man. Basically, human evolution takes place on three different planes, namely physical, mental and spiritual. Yoga is a means of attaining perfect health by maintaining harmony and achieving optimum functioning on all three levels through complete self control. The practice of yoga asanas leads to a well-balanced personality. It improves circulation and energies and stimulates major endocrine glands of the body.

Yogic exercises promote inner health and harmony, and their regular practice helps prevent and cure many common ailments. They also help eliminate tensions, be they physical, mental or emotional. They improve suppleness, grace and posture and keep the spine flexible. They are said to improve appearance and delay old age.

Yoga asanas should be practised only after mastering the techniques with the help of a competent teacher. Asanas should be performed at a leisurely slow-motion pace, maintaining poise and balance. Some of the more important, useful and easy-to-practise asanas which contribute to good health and youthful appearance are described herein in brief:

1. Shavasana (Dead body pose): Lie flat on your back, feet comfortably apart, arms and hands extended about six inches from the body, palms upwards and fingers half-folded. Close your eyes. Begin by consciously and gradually relaxing every part and each muscle of the body: feet, legs, calves, knees, thighs, abdomen, hips, back, hands, arms, chest, shoulders, neck, head and face. Relax yourself completely feeling as if your whole body is lifeless. Now concentrate your mind on breathing rhythmically as slowly and effortlessly as possible. This creates a state of complete relaxation. Remain motionless in this position, relinquishing all responsibilities and worries for 10 to 15 minutes. Discontinue the exercise when your legs grow numb. This asana relaxes the mind and smoothens the nervous system. It should be performed both at the beginning and at the end of the daily round of yogic asanas.

2. Padmasana: Sit erect and stretch your legs out in front of you. Bend one leg to place the foot on the thigh of the other, the sole facing upwards. Similarly, bend the other leg too, so that heels are opposite each other and placed in such a way that they press down on the other side of the groin. Keep your neck, head and spine straight. Place your palms one upon the other, both turned upward and cupped, and rest them on the upturned heels a little below the navel.

Padmasana is good for doing pranayama and meditation. It helps in the treatment of many heart and lung diseases and digestive disorders. It also calms and refreshes the mind.

3. Yogamudra: Sit erect in padmasana. Fold your hands behind your back, holding your left wrist with the right hand. Take

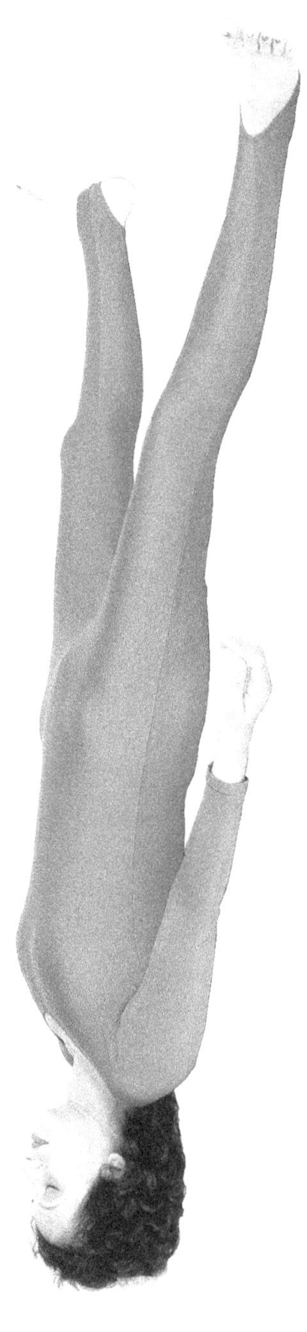

Shavasana

a deep breath. While exhaling, bend forward slowly keeping your hands on your back. Bring your face downwards until your nose and forehead touch the floor. While inhaling, slowly rise back to the upright position. The practice of this asana tones up the nervous system, builds up powerful abdominal muscles and strengthens the pelvic organs. It helps pep up digestion, boosts the appetite and cures constipation.

4. Vajrasana (Pelvic pose): Sit erect and stretch out your legs. Fold your legs back, placing feet on the sides of the buttocks with the soles facing back and upwards. Rest your buttocks on the floor between your heels. The toes of both feet should touch the ground. Now, place your hands on your knees and keep the spine, neck and head straight. This asana can be performed even after meals. It improves the digestion and is beneficial in cases of dyspepsia, constipation, colitis, seminal weakness and stiffness of the legs. It strengthens the hips, thighs, knees, calves, ankles and toes.

5. Uttanpadasana (Leg-lifiting pose): Lie on your back with leg and arms straight, feet together, palms facing downwards, on the floor close to the body. Raise your legs about two feet from the floor without bending your knees. Maintain this pose for some time. Then, lower your legs slowly without bending the knees. This asana is helpful for those suffering from constipation. It strengthens the abdominal muscles and intestinal organs.

6. Bhujangasana (Cobra pose): Lie on your stomach with your legs straight and feet together, toes pointing backwards. Rest your forehead and nose on the ground. Place your palms below the shoulders and your arms by the sides of the chest. Inhale and slowly raise your head, neck, chest and upper abdomen from the navel up. Bend your spine back and arch your back as far as you can, looking upwards. Maintain this position and hold your breath for a few seconds. Exhale, and slowly return to the original position. This asana removes weakness of the abdomen and tones up the reproductive system in women. It exercises the vertebra, back muscles and the spine.

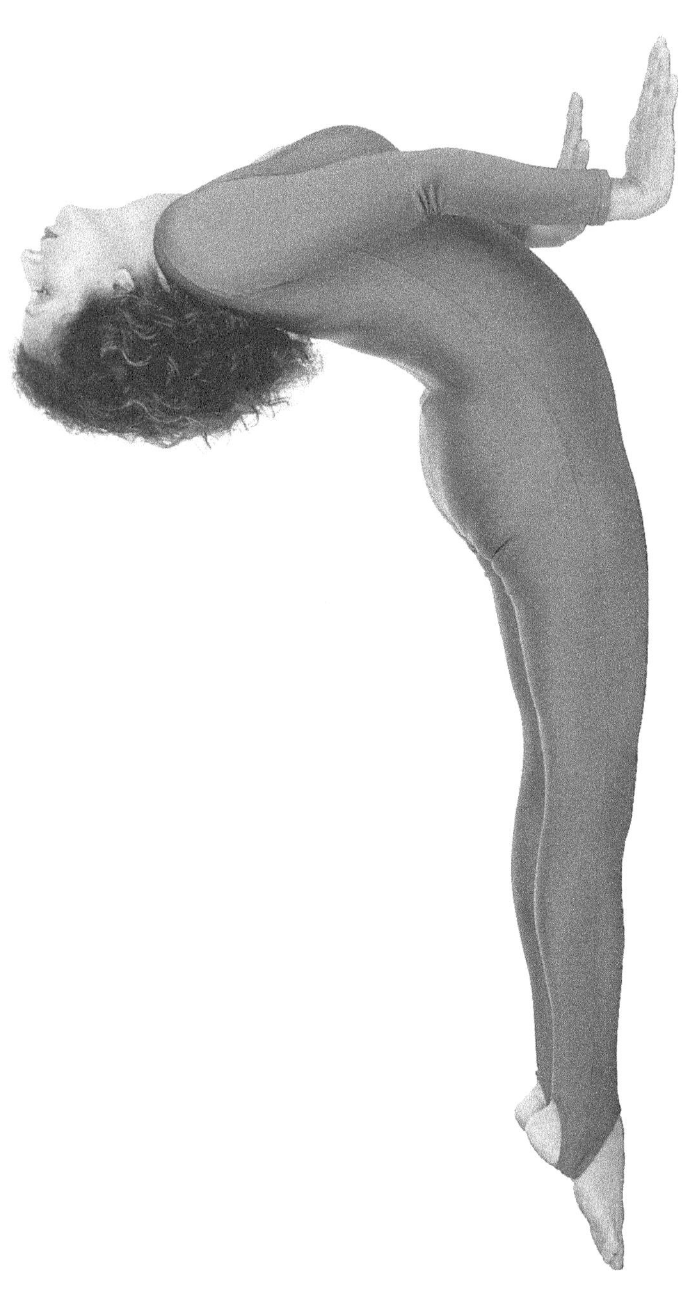

Bhujangasana

7. Shalabhasana (Locust pose): Lie flat on your stomach, with your legs stretched out straight, feet together, chin and nose resting on the ground, looking straight ahead. Move your arms under the body, keeping them straight, fold your hands into fists and place them close to the thighs. Now, raise your legs up, keeping them straight together and stretching them as far back as possible without bending your knees and toes. Hold this position for a few seconds and repeat four or five times. This asana strengthens the whole body, especially the waist, chest, back and neck.

8. Pawanmuktasana (Gas-releasing pose): Lie flat on your back, hands by your side. Fold your legs back, placing your feet flat on the floor; make a fingerlock with your hands and place them a little below the knees. Bring your thighs up near your chest. Exhale and raise head and shoulders and bring your nose between your knees. This is the final position. Maintain this pose for a few seconds and repeat three to five times. Reverse the procedure to get back to the original position.

This asana strengthens the abdominal muscles and internal abdominal organs like the liver, spleen, pancreas and stomach. It helps release excessive gas from the abdomen and relieves flatulence. Persons suffering from constipation should do this exercise in the morning, after drinking lukewarm water to help proper evacuation of the bowels.

9. Chakrasana (Lateral bending pose): Stand straight with your feet and toes together and arms by your sides, palms facing and touching the thighs. Raise one arm laterally above the head with the palm inwards up to shoulder level and palm upwards when the arm rises above the level of your head. Then, bend your trunk and head sideways with the raised arm touching the ear, and sliding the palm of the other hand downwards toward the knee. Keep your knees and elbows straight throughout. Maintain the final pose for a few seconds. Then gradually bring your hand back to the normal position. Repeat the exercise on the other side. This asana

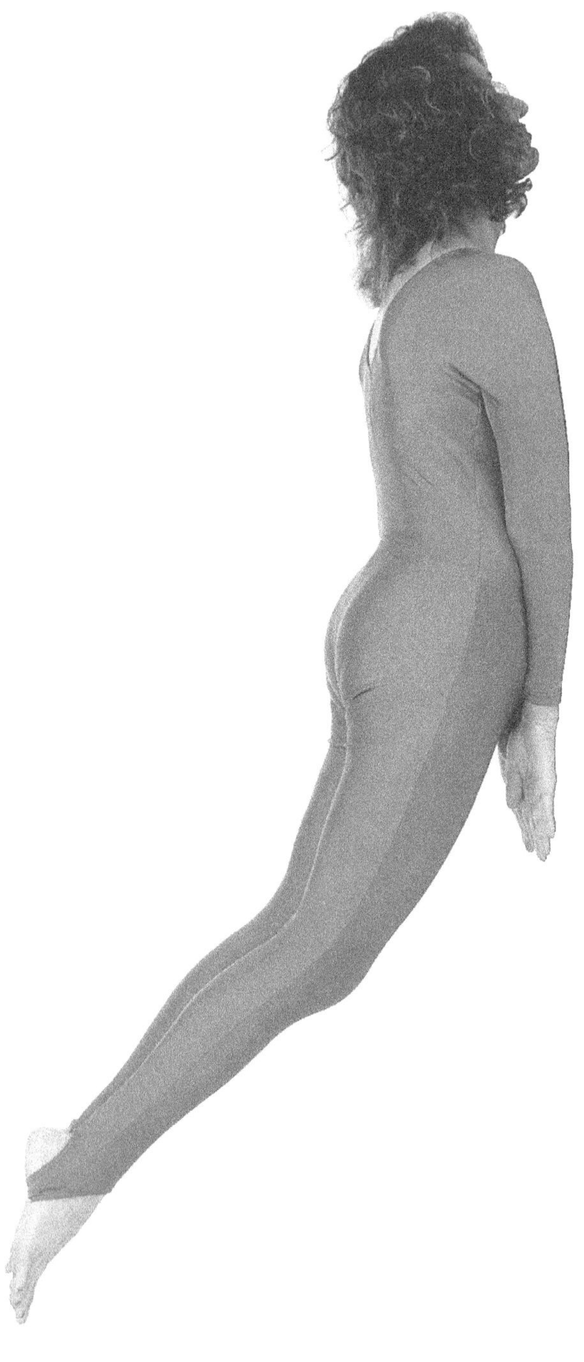

Shalabhasana

induces maximum stretching of the lateral muscles of the body, especially the abdomen. It strengthens the knees, arms and shoulders and increases lung capacity.

10. Vakrasana: Sit erect and stretch legs out. Raise your right knee until your foot rests by the side of the left knee. Place your right hand behind your back without twisting the trunk too much. Then bring your left arm from in front of you over the right knee. Place your left palm on the ground near the heel of your right foot. Push your right knee as far to the left as possible, offering a little resistance to the left arm. Twist your trunk to the right as much as possible. Turn over face to the right over the right shoulder. Release and repeat on the left side.

This asana tones up the spinal and abdominal muscles and nerves and activates the kidneys, intestines, stomach, adrenaline and gonad glands. It relieves cases of constipation and dyspepsia.

11. Vipareetakarani (Inverted action pose): Lie fat on your back, with your feet together and arms by your side. Press your palms down, raising your legs to a perpendicular position without bending the knees. Your palms should touch the waist. Then straighten your legs. The trunk should not make a right angle with the ground but simply an upward slanting position. The chest should not press against the chin but be kept a little away. To return to the ground, bring your legs down slowly, evenly balancing your weight. Through this asana, the muscles of the neck become stronger and blood circulation is improved. The functioning of the cervical nerves, ganglia and the thyroid also gets improved.

12. Sarvagasana (Shoulder stand pose): Lie flat on your back with your arms by the side, palms turned down. Bring your legs up slowly to a 90° angle and then raise the rest of the body by pushing the legs up and resting their weight on the arms. Fix your chin in Jugular Notch, and use your arms and hands to support the body at the hip region. The weight of the body should rest on your head, back and shoulders, your arms being used merely

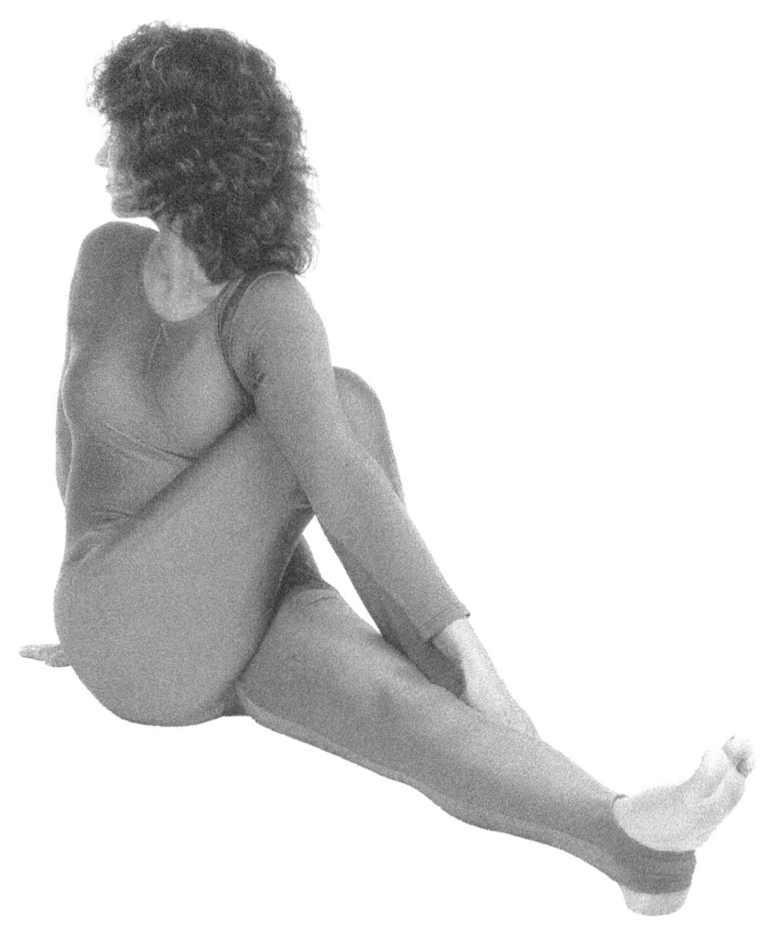

Vakrasana

for balance. The body, legs, hips and trunk should be kept as vertical as possible. Focus your eyes on your big toes. Press your chin against your chest. Hold the pose for one to three minutes. Return to the starting position slowly reversing the procedure.

Sarvagasana helps relieve bronchitis, dyspepsia, varicose veins and peps up the digestion. It stimulates the thyroid and para-thyroid glands, influences the brain, heart and lungs. This asana should not be done by those suffering from high blood pressure, heart disease and eye troubles.

13. Halasana (Plough pose): Lie flat on your back with legs and feet together, arms by your side with fists closed near your thigh. Keeping your legs straight, slowly raise them to angles of 30°, 60° and 90° pausing slightly at each point. Gradually, raise your legs above your head without bending your knees and then move them behind until they touch the floor. Stretch your legs as far as possible so that your chin presses tightly against the chest while your arms remain on the floor as in the original position. Hold the pose from between 10 seconds to three minutes, breathing normally. To return to the starting position slowly reverse the procedure. This asana relieves tension in the back, neck and legs and is beneficial in the treatment of lumbago, spinal rigidity and rheumatism, myalgia, arthritis, sciatica and asthma.

14. Dhanurasana (Bow pose): Lie on your stomach with your chin resting on the ground, arms extended alongside the body with the legs straight. Bend your legs back towards the hips, bring them forward and grasp your ankles. Inhale and raise your thighs, chest and head at the same time. Keep your hands straight. The weight of the body should rest mainly on the navel region. Therefore, arch your spine as much as possible. Exhale and return slowly to the starting position, by reversing the procedure.

Dhanurasana provides good exercise for the arms, shoulders, legs, ankles, back and neck. It also strengthens the spine. It relieves flatulence and constipation and improves the functioning of the

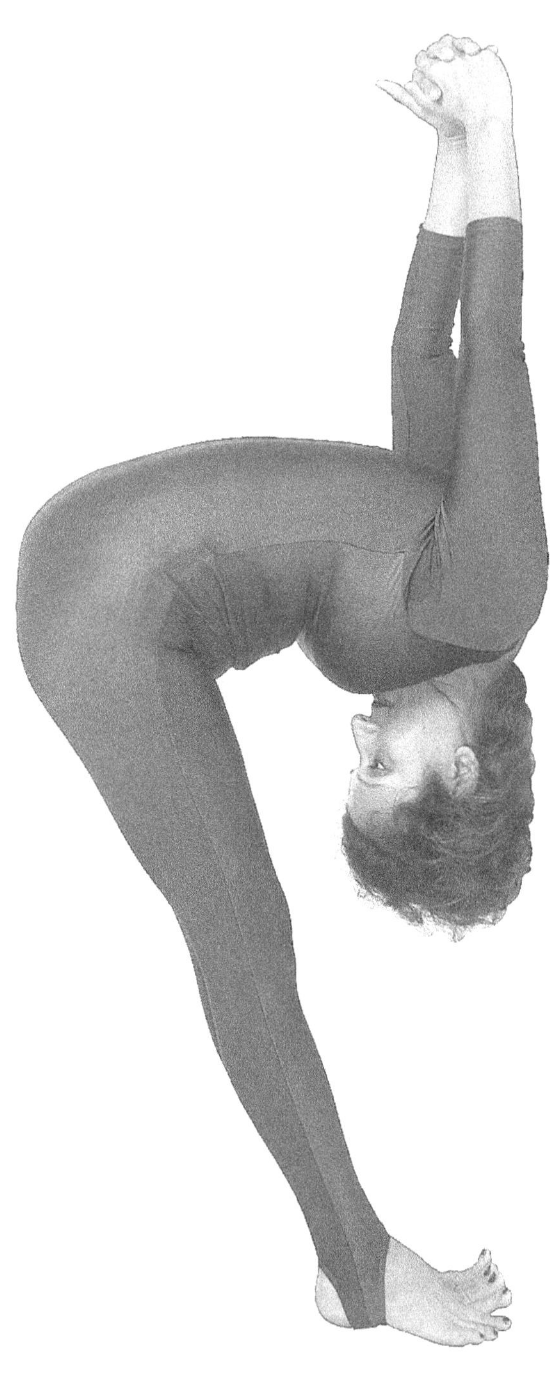

Halasana

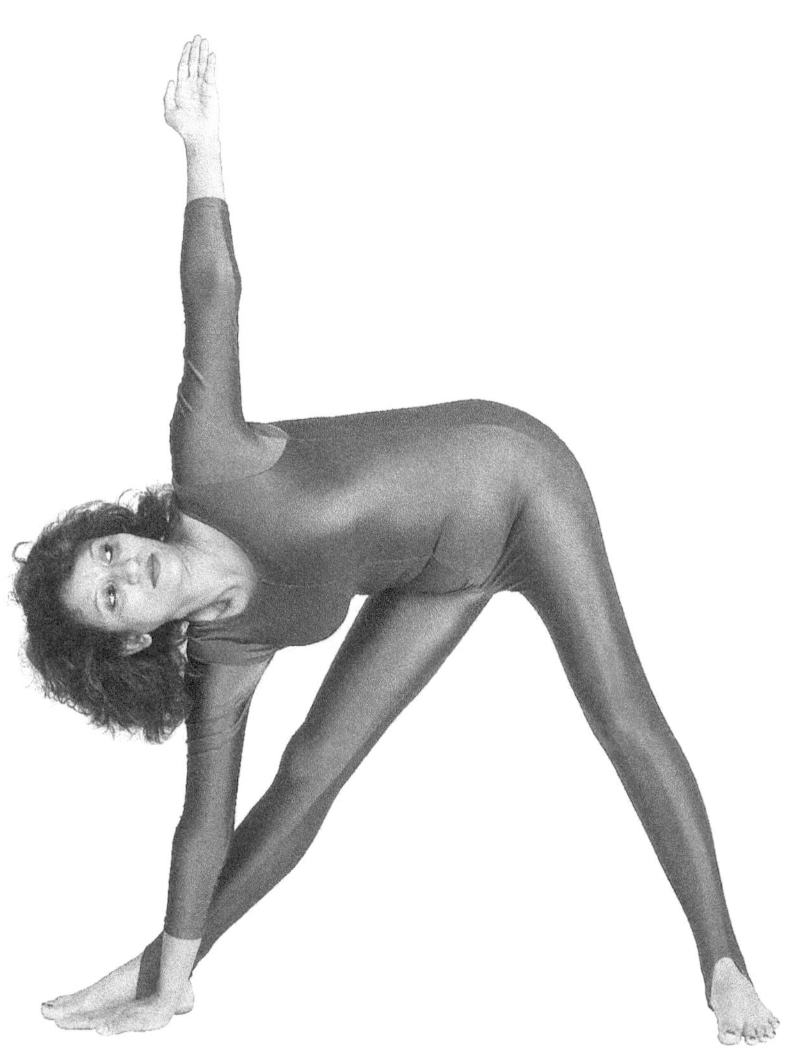

Trikonasana

pancreas and the intestines. It should not be done by those with a weak heart, high blood pressure and ulcers of the stomach and bowels.

15. Paschimottanasana (Posterior stretching pose): Sit erect. Stretch your legs out in front of you, keeping them close to each other. Bend your trunk and head forward from the waist without bending your knees and grasp the big toes with your fingers. Holding your toes, and without bending your knees, rest your forehead on your knees. With practice, the tense muscles become supple enough for this exercise. Old persons and persons whose spine is still should do this asana slowly in the initial stages. The final pose need be maintained only for a few seconds. Return to the starting position gradually.

Paschimottanasana is a good stretching exercise in which the posterior muscles get stretched and relaxed. It relieves sciatica, muscular rheumatism of the back, backache, lumbago and asthmatic attacks. It relieves one of constipation, dyspepsia and other abdominal disorders.

16. Trikonasana (Triangle pose): Stand erect with your legs apart. Stretch your arms up to shoulder level. Bend your trunk forwards and twist to the left, looking upwards and keeping your left arm forwards and raised at an angle of 90. Place your right palm on your left foot without bending the knees. Maintain this pose for a few seconds. Then straighten up and return to the normal position. Repeat the procedure on the other side. Trikonasana is an all-round stretching exercise. It keeps the spinal column flexible and reduces the fat on the lateral side of the body. Besides, it stimulates the adrenal glands and tones up the abdominal and pelvic organs.

Yoga asanas should be practised on empty stomach. Morning is the best period. The place should be airy and open. All asanas should be performed on a clean mat, a carpet or a blanket covered with a cotton sheet. Clothing should be light and loose-fitting to allow free movements of the limbs. The mind should be kept off all disturbances and tensions. Regularity and punctuality in practising yogic exercises is essential.

CHAPTER 8

Importance of Rest, Relaxation and Meditation in Old Age

Physical and mental rest, adequate sleep, relaxation and meditation are as important as exercise in slowing the ageing process. Rest means the absence of effort. It aims at counterbalancing work in a physiological sense. Relaxation is rest after effort or conscious rest after conscious effort.

Sleep is a periodic rest of the body which is absolutely essential for its efficient functioning. It has been called "most cheering restorative of tired bodies." It is the indispensable condition to the recuperation of energy. A person goes to bed fatigued and gets up refreshed. Sleep repairs the wear and tear of the body and mind incurred during waking hours. Nothing is so restorative to the nerves as sound and uninterrupted sleep.

Two-thirds of the total weight of the body consists of the life-giving element, oxygen. Work consumes oxygen and reduces the body's store of this wonderful element. As the oxygen diminishes, the vital activities wane. Tissue waste, the consumption of the entire physical structure, from brain to cuticle, takes place during working hours. Sleep is the only time, when reparative processes, which may overcome all this waste, can occur. Studies have shown that the average amount of sleep needed to feel well rested is seven and a half hours. However, individual needs may vary from six to nine hours.

Loss of sleep exerts seriously detrimental effects upon the nervous system. Long periods of wakefulness may cause profound psychological changes such as loss of memory, irritability, hallucination, even schizophrenic manifestations.

Unpleasant situation at bed time such as arguments, quarrels, watching a horror movie, listening to loud music, which would create anxiety, fear, excitement and worries, should be avoided. Such situation stimulate the cerebral cortex and tend to keep one awake. The sleeping place should be well ventilated, with balanced temperature and free from noises. The bed should be neither too hard, nor too soft, but comfortable. The pillow should not be too hard or too high. The bed clothes should be loose-fitting and light coloured. Another important rule is not to eat heavy food shortly before bed time.

It is essential for the elderly to learn how to relax physically and mentally. In relaxation, the muscles work more efficiently. Fatigue is also completely relieved in a very short time as the venous blood circulation is promoted throughout the body. The best method of relaxation is to practise savasana or 'The dead pose.' The procedure for practising this asana has been explained in the previous chapter.

Another method of relaxation, mentioned by Indira Devi in her book *Forever Young, Forever Healthy*, is as follows: Lie down on a carpet and stretch. Stretch your arms way back over your head and stretch your legs, making the whole body as stiff as you can. Then abruptly drop your hands down alongside of you and relax the whole body. With eyes closed, concentrate first on the tip of your toes and try to relax them. Imagine that your feet, legs and thighs are being gradually plunged into pleasantly warm water and all the muscles are becoming relaxed. Next, relax your back, spine and shoulders; then your arms, hands and finger-tips. Let your chin drop so that the muscles of your face relax as well. And, now, imagine that your body is getting heavier and heavier so heavy that it sinks into the carpet and you no longer feel its weight. Remain like this for a few minutes completely relaxed and completely at ease.

Now visualise yourself as a cloud — very light and carefree just floating in the vast blue sky. After a while, dismiss this vision. Then try to keep your mind as blank as possible. Imagine yourself sinking into complete oblivion. You are now relaxed, and feel like a light cloud floating in the sky. Before getting up, stretch and yawn.

Older people should learn to avoid nerve tensions. Whenever you have a chance during the day, arrange to sit quietly and relax every muscle of your body. If you are alone, you can keep your eyes closed and think about the omnipresence and omnipotence of the creator, and try to feel your inner mind merging or uniting with the all-pervading divine mind essence.

The older people should also meditate frequently and they should explore and develop their spiritual interests. The state of meditation or dhyana is achieved when the mind is trained to concentrate on an outer or inner object, long enough for all distractions to be eliminated, and when the stream of thoughts flows in a single direction without interruption. The body is silently resting in this state. The only sign of life is breathing. The hypothalamus recharges its energy during meditation.

Meditation helps eliminate emotional conflict, inner discord and psychological tension. It completely purifies the mind and frees it from unconscious obstructions. The most common method consists in concentrating one's attention on an object of personal value or a universal symbol.

Each person, according to his faith, usually chooses an elevated thought or spiritual symbol upon which he prefers to meditate.

It is essential to adopt a comfortable and firm posture, otherwise meditation will not be possible. To adopt a firm posture

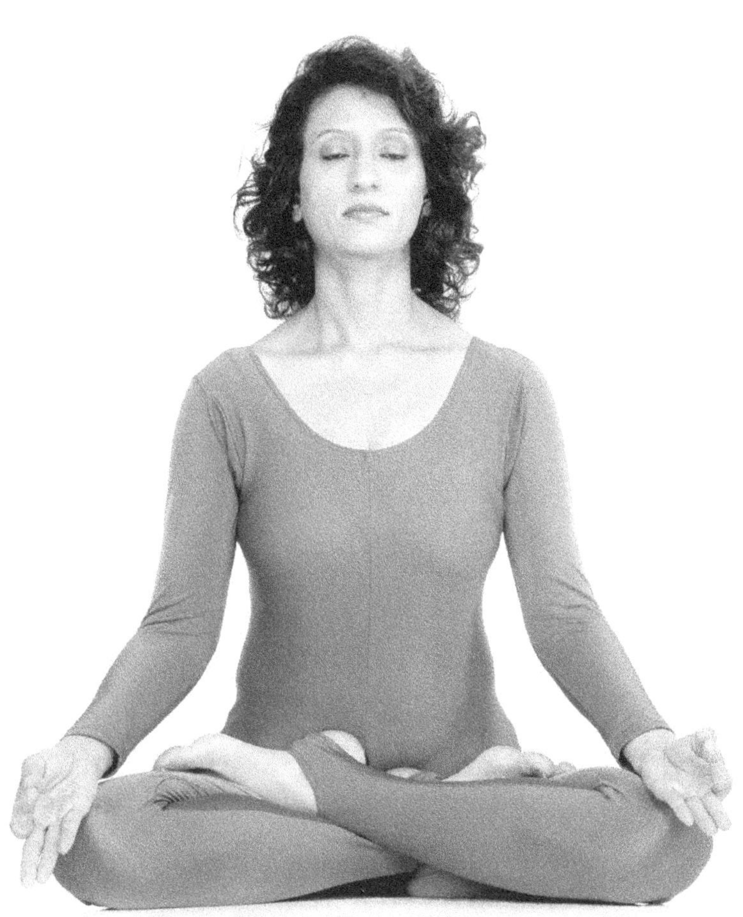

Meditation

means to hold oneself in such a way that one is conscious of the body. The slightest discomfort in such a posture will prove a constant distraction to the mind; one should therefore choose the position that allows one to remain still for a long time without feeling discomfort. The spine and head should be kept very straight, but without being strained. Padmasana is considered to be the ideal posture for practising meditation. The procedure for this asana has been explained in the previous chapter.

CHAPTER 9

Weight Control for Healthy Old Age

Proper weight control is of utmost importance in old age. It is seen that obesity is one of the most common nutritional disorders in the elderly. It has in general grown proportionate to the growth of junk foods. Obesity may be described as a bodily condition characterised by excessive deposition or storage of fat in adipose tissue. It usually results from consumption of food in excess of physiological needs. Some gain in fat is expected as we age. About one kg of weight gain every decade after the age of 30 is considered reasonable. Excess weight gain, however, is a cause for great concern in old age.

Obesity is generally assessed by relating patients' weight to charts of standard weight prevailing in different parts of the world. They are then categorised 10, 20 or 30 per cent overweight. Gross obesity is, however, uncommon in the elderly because persons who are morbidly obese are more likely to die earlier due to complications of their obesity.

Obesity is a serious health hazard as the extra fat puts a strain on the heart, kidneys and liver as well as the large weight-bearing joints such as the hips, knees and ankles, which ultimately shortens the life span. It has been aptly said, 'the longer the belt, the shorter the life.' Overweight elderly persons are susceptible to several diseases like accidents, coronary thrombosis, heart failure, high blood pressure, diabetes, arthritis, gout, varicose veins and liver and gallbladder disorders.

There are certain distinguishing features of obesity in the elderly. The most important is the sex difference. Obesity, particularly the severe type, is mostly confined to the female. This is because it is responsible for increased mortality in the elderly male and hence the lower prevalence in them. Another important feature of obesity in the elderly is that it rarely occurs for the first time in older persons. Hence, obese older persons usually suffer from this disease from an earlier age.

Osteoarthritis of the major weight-bearing joints (hips, knees) is an inevitable result of long-standing obesity. This severely restricts the already impaired mobility of older patients. Energy expenditure is reduced and the disease becomes severe.

Chronic pains may lead to ingestion of large amounts of analgesic which can result in significant gastrointestinal blood loss and the development of iron-deficiency anaemia.

The main cause of obesity, most often, is overeating, that is, the intake of calories beyond the body's energy requirement. Recent studies have, however, shown that reduced physical activity is also a major functional abnormality in obese persons. There has also been in recent times, an increasing awareness of psychological aspects of obesity. Older persons who are generally bored, unhappy, lonely or unloved, those who are discontented with their families, or social or financial standing, usually tend to overeat as eating is a pleasure and solace to them.

Treatment

Many strategies for losing weight have been planned and tried over years because, as a rule, losing weight and keeping the weight off are extremely difficult. This is particularly true for those, individuals who are 25% or more overweight.

A suitably planned course of dietary treatment, in conjunction with suitable exercise and other measures for promoting elimination, is the only scientific way of dealing with obesity. The chief consideration in this treatment should be the balanced selection of foods which provide the maximum essential nutrients with the least number of calories, ranging from 1,100 to 1,200.

To begin with, the patient should undertake a juice fast for seven to 10 days. Juices of lemon, grapefruit, orange, pineapple, cabbage and carrot may be taken during this period. Long juice fast up to 40 days can also be undertaken, but only under expert guidance and supervision. In the alternative, short juice fasts should be repeated at regular intervals of two months or so till the desired reduction in weight is achieved.

After the juice fast, the patient should spend a further four or five days on an all-fruit diet, taking three meals of fresh juicy fruits, such as oranges, grapefruit, pineapple and papaya. Thereafter, he may gradually embark upon a low-calorie well-balanced diet of three basic food groups, namely (i) seeds, nuts and grains, (ii) vegetable and (iii) fruits, with emphasis on raw fruits, vegetables and fresh juices.

The foods which should be drastically curtailed or altogether avoided are high-fat substances such as butter, cheese, chocolate, cream, ice-cream, fat meats, fried foods and gravies; high carbohydrate foods like bread, candy, cake, cookies, cereal products, legumes, potatoes, honey, sugar, syrup and rich puddings; beverages such as all-fountain drinks and alcoholic drinks.

Fasting on honey-lime juice water is highly beneficial in the treatment of obesity without the loss of energy and appetite. In this mode of treatment, one spoon of fresh honey should be mixed with a juice of half a lime in a glass of lukewarm water and taken at regular intervals.

Cabbage is considered to be an effective home remedy for obesity. This vegetable contains a valuable content called tetanic acid which inhibits the conversion of sugar and other carbohydrates

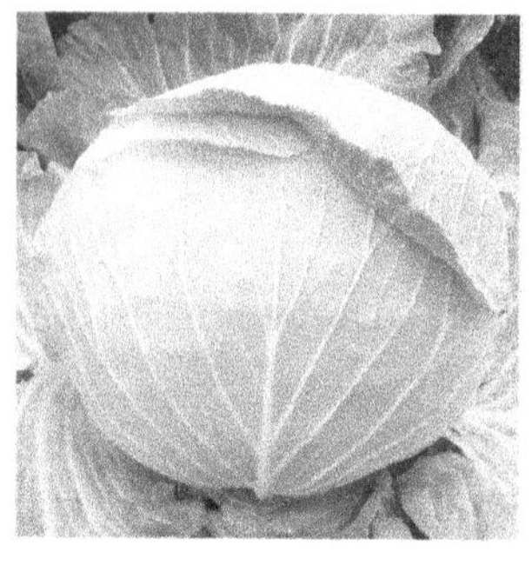

into fat. Hence, it is of great value in weight reduction. A helping of cabbage salad would be the simplest way to stay slim, a painless way of dieting.

Along with dietetic treatment, the patient should adopt all other natural methods of reducing weight. Exercise is an important part of weight reduction plan. It helps to use up calories stored in body fat and relieves tension, besides toning up the muscles of the body. Walking is the best exercise to begin with and may be followed by running, swimming, rowing and other outdoor sports.

Certain yogic asanas are highly beneficial. They not only break up or re-distribute fatty deposits and help slimming, but also strengthen the flabby areas. These asanas include bhujangasana, shalabhasana, chakrasana, vajrasana, yogamudra and trikonasana. They work on the glands, improve circulation, strengthen many weak areas and induce deep breathing which helps to melt off excess fat gradually.

CHAPTER 10

Thirty Useful Tips for Better Living

Elderly persons should take certain precautionary measures to make old age happy, safe and comfortable. Herein are given 30 useful tips which the elderly can follow with great advantage:

1. Develop a positive outlook towards changed style of living. Since the process of ageing is inevitable, accept old age gracefully and learn to enjoy the remaining years of life.
2. Cultivate healthy habits. Eat natural foods and undertake moderate exercises, specially walking and yogic practices. Avoid smoking and drinking.
3. Eat less. Calorie restriction can prevent age-related diseases and slow down ageing process.
4. Develop spiritual outlook and pray regularly as prayer strengthens the body and prolongs life.
5. Take adequate rest, relax as often as possible, and sleep well. An afternoon nap can boost your life span as well as your performance.
6. Laugh as often as possible as laughter exercises the body, relaxes muscle tension, improves circulation and builds up body resistance.
7. Do not brood over the past events, nor worry about the

future events, but concentrate on present happenings around you.

8. Adjust your needs to suit the purse and learn to live like a common man.
9. Keep yourself occupied with some useful pursuits of your choice which may bring some money. Also cultivate some useful hobbies like music, painting and gardening.
10. You can stay active and productive by participating in community work like better environment projects, adult literacy programme, taking interest in civil facilities, voluntary service at old-age homes and handicapped centres and consumer protection work.
11. Avoid squatting on the floor in the house or elsewhere as it may cause pain in the groins and joints of legs. Sit on a chair, bench, sofa or firm stool with your legs on the floor. Adopt a posture in which the back remains erect.
12. Keep a small torch handy near the pillow at night, so that when you get up to answer nature's call, you can easily locate the bathroom without difficulty and without disturbing others in their sleep.
13. Take bath in a sitting position preferably on a small stool. Never bathe in a standing position as the weight of the body is on the legs and there is every possibility of slippage because the bathroom floor has a lot of soap lather and other oily substances which make it slippery. Accidents usually take place in the bathroom.
14. Take time over your appearance and grooming. Brush the hair and clip the nails. Wear neatly-pressed clothes as they are positive signs of self-esteem. Use clean and somewhat loose clothes and always wear a smile
15. Wear well-fitting shoes or slippers with non-slip soles. Avoid long shoelaces, which can get untied easily and cause you to trip.

16. Never walk around with glasses on your nose, if they are meant for reading only. Take them off while walking about.
17. Store frequently-used items in places where you can reach them easily. Avoid climbing on the chairs or stools unnecessarily. Climb only if you must, but ensure that you have a sturdy and stable ladder or chair or stool.
18. While walking on the road, always keep to the extreme right side of the road which is relatively safe for pedestrians This will help prevent accidents from speeding vehicles.
19. Also keep your pace somewhat slow so that you can pause for a while when a speeding vehicle passes by.
20. If you have to cross the road, take all precautions and cross only when you consider it very safe. Do not hesitate to take the help of a fellow pedestrian, younger than you, in crossing a busy road.
21. Do not think or brood over some issue while walking or crossing the road. Keep all your attention on the road and the traffic only.
22. Take a walk early in the morning, if possible, when there is much less traffic on the road and the atmosphere is also less polluted.
23. If you have to climb, take the support of the railing with one hand and keep your attention on placing your feet carefully and firmly on the steps of the staircase. A little carelessness in placing a foot on the steps may cause slippage and result in an accident.
24. Travel light, when you travel by train, bus, boat, plane, or in your own car. Take no more luggage than you are able to carry on your own.
25. Continue to take interest in your sex life. Physical closeness and warmth are important.

26. Spend a lot more time with your spouse. Give opportunity to each other for independent activities and share the domestic work with your spouse.
27. Make a formal will, if you have not done so already. If necessary, inform a close relative or friend of its contents and its location.
28. If you are living with your son or daughter, schedule your activities to suit their convenience. A little thoughtfulness goes a long way in maintaining a congenial atmosphere.
29. Give advice to your children only when asked and that too sparingly. That way, you ensure that you will be heeded.
30. Be realistic in your expectations of your adult children. Accept the way they conduct their lives and their career choices.

SECTION II

NERVOUS SYSTEM AND MENTAL DISODERS

CHAPTER 11

Amnesia

Brain

Investigations conducted in several laboratories show that brain does not necessarily corrode with age, so long as it is free of actual disease. Researches over the past several years have shown that the human brain can grow in a variety of ways in a surprising manner, even in advanced old age. Neuroscientist Robert Terry of the University of California, has shown that the brain cells called neurons, which are responsible for processing information, do not really die off with age, they merely shrink. And although these smaller neurons do not function as well as larger ones, Terry thinks they might be regrown or retrained to work normally.

There is a concern among older people that if they do not constantly exercise their memory cells they may vanish by sheer disuse. Most people lose memory and thus suffer from amnesia because they constantly worry about losing it. Different types and degrees of amnesia are found in old age. Recent memory is far less efficient in the elderly, although long-term memory still functions well.

Symptoms

The most common form of amnesia in the elderly is verbal amnesia. In this condition, the patient forgets words and names.

A very uncommon form of amnesia is temporary loss of memory, in which a person even forgets his own identity, including his name, age, family background and any recollection of the past. In case of poor memory caused by brain weakness, the patient may suffer from mild headache, intolerance to noise and inability to concentrate.

Causes

The main cause of amnesia in older persons is the impairment of mental faculties. Other causes are impairment of brain cells due to diseases affecting them directly or indirectly through a poor blood supply due to circulatory diseases. Poor memory also results from dullness of intellect and weakness of brain. Many cases are, however, largely psychological in origin, caused by anxiety, neurosis, resulting from lack of attention in persons obsessed with their own problems.

According to Dr. Barry Gordon, a behavioural neurologist and Head of the division of Cognitive Neurology at Johns Hopkins University School of Medicine in Baltimore, Maryland, excessive consumption of alcohol could be a cause of memory loss in some people since it could damage nerve cells, especially if taken with prescription drugs like tranquilizers, antidepressants or antacids. The extent of daily use and number of years in use of the drugs plays a part. People do not necessarily remember more accurately under hypnosis; they may remember more true facts but they are also likely to 'recall' many untrue 'memories' as well.

Treatment

Diet is of utmost importance in the treatment of amnesia, it should be so arranged as to provide all essential nutrients as even a single nutritional deficiency can cause anxiety neurosis in susceptible people. Older persons suffering from amnesia should avoid tea, coffee, alcohol, chocolate and cola, all white flour products, sugar, food colourings, chemical additives, white rice and strong condiments.

The diet should be restricted to three meals. Fruits can be taken in the morning for breakfast with milk and a handful of nuts and seeds. Lunch may consist of steamed vegetables, whole wheat chapattis and a glass of buttermilk. For dinner, green vegetables salad and all available sprouts such as alfalfa seeds and mung beans, cottage cheese or a glass of buttermilk would be ideal. The patient should take liberally phosphorus-rich foods like cereals, pulses, nuts, fruit juices and milk. Cow's milk is specially beneficial and the patient should take as much of this milk as he can safely digest.

Certain home remedies have been found beneficial in the treatment of amnesia. The most remarkable of these is the use of the herb brahmi booti, botanically known as Bacopa scrophulariaceae. About seven grams of this herb should be dried in the shade and ground in water, along with seven kernels of almond and four and half decigrams of pepper, strained and sweetened with honey. This should be drunk every morning for a fortnight on an empty stomach.

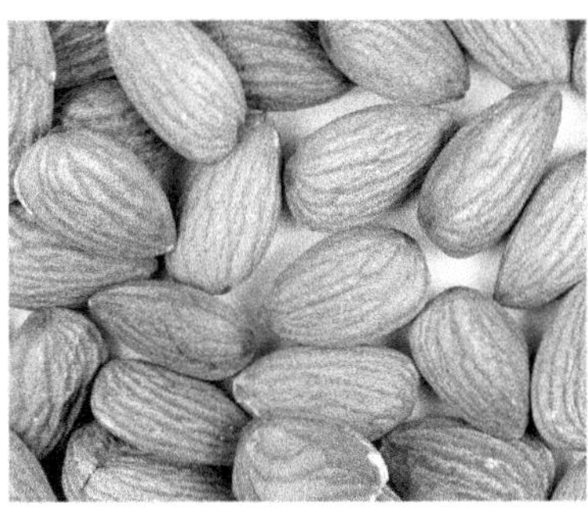

Almond (badam) is very valuable in poor memory caused by brain weakness. It contains unique properties to remove brain debility and to strengthen it. This dry fruit preserves the vitality of the brain and cures ailments originating from nervous disorders. Almonds should be immersed in water for an hour or so and their upper red coating removed. They should then be made into a fine paste by rubbing them on a stone slab with sandalwood and taken mixed with butter or alone. Inhaling 10 to 15 drops of almond oil through the nose is also beneficial in the treatment of brain weakness.

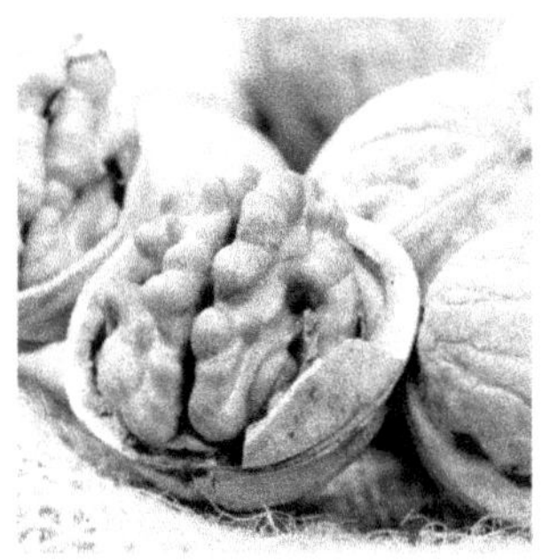

Walnut (akhrot) is another unique dry fruit valuable in brain weakness. Its value will be enhanced if it is taken with fgs or raisins. If it is intended to be consumed alone, about 20 grams of walnuts should be taken every day.

All the fruits, which are rich in phosphorus, are valuable in amnesia, as they invigorate the brain cells and tissues. The fruits are figs, grapes, dates, oranges, besides almond, walnut and apple. Their use is highly beneficial in loss of memory due to brain debility.

A pinch of finely ground pepper (gol mirch), mixed with honey, is also beneficial in the treatment of this condition. It should be taken both in the morning and evening.

The patient must gain control over his nervous system and channelise his mental and emotional activities into restful harmonious vibrations. This can be achieved by proper rest and sleep. He must also learn the art of scientific relaxation and meditation. The procedure for practising relaxation and meditation has been explained in Chapter 8 under Section I.

CHAPTER 12

Depression

Hippocrates (460 - 370 B.C.), the father of medicine, included depression in his classification of mental illness. It has been called 'the common cold of psychiatry.' It is the most prevalent of all the emotional disorders. It may vary from feelings of slight sadness to utter misery and dejection. It is the most unpleasant experience a person can endure and is far more difficult to cope with than a physical ailment.

There is a marked increase in the incidence of depression in old age. The percentage of incidence rises progressively with age as well as its tendency to recurrence. This explains the high suicide rate in men over 60 years. More people over 60 make successful suicide attempts than at any other stage of life.

In many elderly patients, depression is severe and is accompanied by apathy or agitation. They commonly have ideas of guilt or delusions about their physical illness, poverty and unworthiness. Other older persons may suffer from anxiety. Suicide is the distinct risk common in both the types. Their talk of suicide should, therefore be taken seriously by their family members.

Symptoms

The most prominent symptoms of depression are feelings of acute sense of loss and inexplicable sadness, loss of energy and loss of interest. The patient feels tired and lacks interest in the world around him. He may suffer from sleep disturbances such as difficulty in getting off to sleep at night, nightmares and repeated waking from midnight onwards. He often has oppressive feeling and self-absorption. Other symptoms of depression are loss of appetite, giddiness, itching, nausea, agitation, irritability, impotence or frigidity, constipation, aches and pains all over the body, lack of concentration and lack of power of decision. Cases of severe depression may be characterised by low body temperature, low blood pressure, hot flushes and shivering. The external manifestations represent a cry for help from the tormented mind of the depressed person.

Causes

Depleted functioning of the adrenal glands is one of the main causes of mental depression. Irregular diet habits causes digestive problems and lead to the assimilation of fats. An excess of carbohydrates like cereals, white sugar, coffee, tea, chocolates and comparatively less quantities of vegetables and fruits in the diet may result in indigestion. This leads to formation of gases in the digestive tract, causing compression over the diaphragm, in the region of the heart and lungs. Consequently, the supply of oxygen to the tissues is reduced. This raises the carbon dioxide level and results in general depression.

The excessive and indiscriminate use of drugs also leads to faulty assimilation of vitamins and minerals by the body and ultimately causes depression. Diabetes, low blood sugar and weakness of the liver resulting from the use of refined processed foods, fried foods and an excessive intake of fats may also lead to depression.

Treatment

The treatment of depression with anti-depression drugs may provide temporary relief but have harmful side-effects and do not remove the causes. The harmful side-effects include gross liver damage, hypersensitivity, insomnia, hallucinations, a confused state, convulsions, a fall in blood pressure which may cause headaches and dizziness, blurred vision and urine retention. The plan of action in nature cure for the treatment of depression consists of regulating the diet, physical exercise, scientific relaxation and meditation.

Diet plays a vital role in the mental health of a person. Even a single nutritional deficiency can cause depression in susceptible people. Dr. Priscilla, associate clinical professor at the University of California, prescribes nutritional therapy to build up brain chemicals, such as serotonin and norepinephrine, that effect mood and are often lacking in depressed people. She recommends eating foods rich in B vitamins, such as whole grains, green vegetables, eggs and fish.

In the last two decades, a number of studies have shown that some foods influence the production of brain chemicals that are directly involved in determining our mood, mental energy, performance and behaviour. Some of the most important 'good mood' foods are whole grain bread, bananas, oranges and grapefruits. Whole grain bread is rich in amino acid tryptophan. Once it enters the brain, this amino acid boosts levels of serotonin, the soothing, mood-elevating brain chemical.

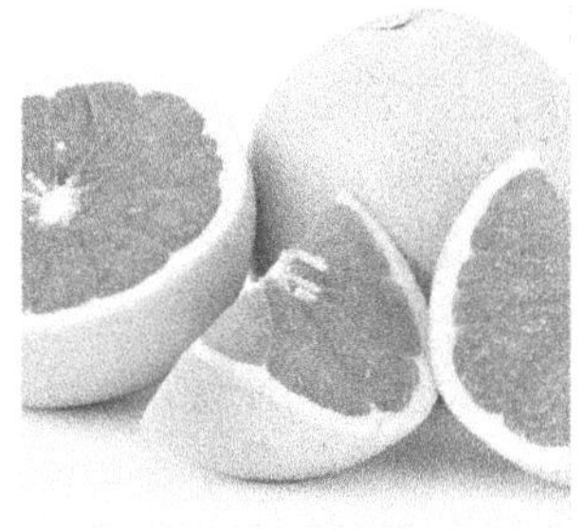

As a rich source of magnesium, bananas have been found beneficial in the treatment of depression. Researchers have shown that increased magnesium intake results in less anxiety and better sleep. Other rich sources of magnesium are nuts, beans and leafy green vegetables. Vitamin C-rich fruits like oranges and grapefruits have also been found valuable in depression. Researchers have proved that even a small deficiency in Vitamin C can leave a person irritable and depressed. A lack of Vitamin C-rich foods also inhibits the body's ability to absorb the iron it needs to fight fatigue.

The older persons suffering from depression should avoid strong tea, coffee, alcoholic beverages, soft drinks, all white flour products, white sugar, food colourings, chemical additives and strong condiments. Their diet should be based on three basic food groups, namely seeds, nuts and grains, vegetables and fruits. The emphasis should be on fresh fruits, raw vegetables, salad, whole grain cereals and fresh fruit and vegetable juices.

Home Remedies

Certain home remedies have been found beneficial in the treatment of depression. The most important of these is the use of apple (seb). The various chemical substances present in this fruit, such as Vitamin B1, phosphorus and potassium help the synthesis of glutamic acid, which controls the wear and tear of nerve cells. Atleast one fruit should be eaten daily with milk and honey. This will act as a very effective nerve tonic and recharge the nerves with new energy and life. The cashewnut (Kaju) is another valuable remedy for general depression and nervous weakness. It is rich in vitamins of B group, especially thiamine and therefore useful in stimulating appetite and nervous system. It is also rich in riboflavin which keeps the body active, gay and energetic.

The use of root of asparagus (shatawar) has been found beneficial in the treatment of depression. It is highly nutritious and is used as a herbal medicine for mental disorders. It is a good tonic for the brain and nerves. Cardamom (illaichi) has proved useful in depression. Powdered seeds should be boiled in water and tea prepared in the usual way. It gives a very pleasing aroma to tea

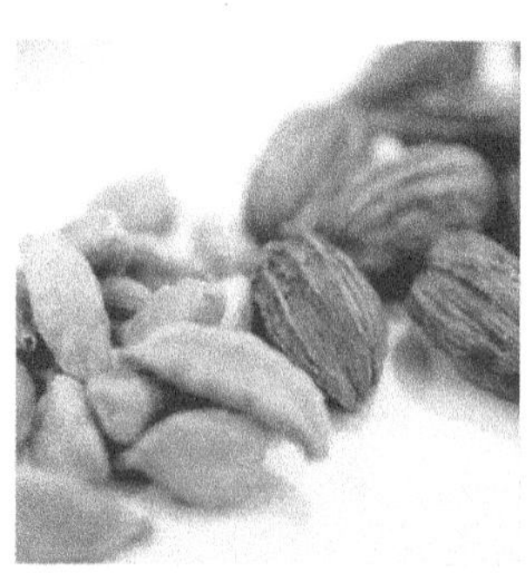

which can be used as a medicine in the treatment of this condition.

The herb lemon balm (billilotan) has been used successfully in the treatment of mental depression. It assists brain fatigue, lifts the heart from depression and raises the spirits. A cold infusion of the balm taken freely is reputed to be excellent for its calming influence on the nerves. About 30 grams of the herb should be placed in half a litre of cold water and allowed to stand for 12 hours. The infusion should then be strained and taken in small doses throughout the day. Roses (gulab) have also been found useful in depression. An infusion of rose petals should be used occasionally, instead of the usual tea and coffee for treating this condition.

Activity and Exercise

The depressive mood can be overcome by activity. Those who are depressed will forget their misery by doing something. The pleasure of achievement overcomes the distress of misery.

Exercise also plays an important role in the treatment of depression. It keeps the body physically and mentally fit and provides recreation and mental relaxation. It is nature's best tranquiliser. Exercise changes the levels of hormones in blood, elevates beta-endorphins and improves the function of the automatic nervous system. It gives a feeling of accomplishment and thus reduces sense of helplessness. Some form of active exercise must be undertaken every day at a regular hour. Yogic asanas such as vakrasana, bhujangasana, shalabhasana, halasana, paschimotanasana, sarvangasana and shavasana are beneficial in the treatment of depression.

Adequate rest, relaxation and meditation are also essential to overcome feelings of depression and to gain control over the nervous system. The patient should have sufficient sleep under right condition. He should also relax and meditate as often as possible. This will go a long way in curing depression. The methods for relaxation and meditation have been explained in Chapter 9 under Section I.

CHAPTER 13

Stroke

Neurological diseases are quite common in old age. A wide variety of age changes takes place in the nervous system. These changes include loss of vibration, sense, tendon reflexes in the legs and irregularity and contraction of the pupils.

Stroke is one of the most serious nervous system diseases prevalent in old age. It is an important cause of disability and a major contributor to mortality in old age. The incidence of this disease rises from under 0.25 per 1000 per annum in the 34-44 age group to 20 in the 75-84 decade. Mortality rate also rises with age. Overall prevalence rates have been estimated at 7-12 per 1000 but in those aged 65 years and over, its prevalence rises to 50-70 per 1000.

Also known as apoplexy, stroke is a sudden acute disturbance of brain function of vascular origin. It may result in loss of consciousness, paralysis or death.

Symptoms

Usually, the first sign of stroke is dizziness, followed by nausea and vomitting, and later by weakness of the body. The patient may complain of a severe headache, and may even have a convulsion, or pass into a coma from which he cannot be aroused for some time. He may be completely paralysed on one side and may not be able to speak. He may be mentally alert, but for some time, he may not be able to recall the actual words he wants to use.

Many strokes occur suddenly and tend to clear after a few hours. In more serious cases, the patient may remain in a deep coma for several days. He may have a fever, a rapid pulse and difficult breathing. This condition may arise due to haemorrhage of the brain, if the coma lasts for more than six hours and the patient passes periods of convulsions with stiffness in the neck, and his eyes are turned sharply toward the paralysed side. A severe haemorrhage may prove fatal in two or three days, especially if the patient has a high fever with a rapid pulse.

Most patients recover, if the stroke is due to thrombosis or if only a small vessel is involved. Many of them may not even lose consciousness, but the weakness or paralysis may continue for a long time. There may also be some permanent disability, even with the best of care.

Causes

The brain is a delicate organ requiring a constant supply of blood. A stroke occurs when one of the vessels leading to a portion of the brain becomes blocked by a blood clot. This may be due to inflammation, arteriosclerosis, or the presence of a clot or embolus from the heart. Occasionally, one of the vessels leading to the brain may rupture because of a small aneurysm or enlargement in the wall of the vessel. This will cause a serious haemorrhage. A sudden rise in blood pressure caused by emotions like anger may rupture the aneurysm. Most strokes are due to thrombosis, or clotting of blood within the vessel. When this happens, that portion of the brain becomes necrotic and dies.

Treatment

Good nursing care is of utmost importance, especially during the acute stage. The patient should be made to rest in bed, and he should be turned frequently from side to side to prevent development of pressure sores. Cold compresses may be applied to the head to relieve pain. The patient should be protected from visitors and all forms of excitement. He should not return to work for several months.

The most important factor in treating this disease is fasting. The patient should fast for the first few days and he should be given only water to drink, if he can take it. Thereafter, he may be given orange juice and water. The fast should be continued till the severity of the stroke has passed off. He can then be allowed to take fresh fruits such as orange, apple, pineapple, pear, grapes, peach and papaya. The diet can be extended to include fresh and unboiled milk, and as convalescence progresses, the fruit and milk diet can be gradually followed by a well-balanced diet consisting of seeds, nuts and grains, fruits and vegetables. The emphasis should be on fresh fruits and raw vegetable salads, fruits and vegetable juices. The bowels should be cleansed twice daily with warm-water enema for the first two or three days, and then daily until the bowels begin to function of their own accord.

The patient should be encouraged to use the paralysed limbs and move all the joints several times daily. The paralysed muscles should be gently massaged. As soon as possible, the patient should come out of bed and walk around the room.

When he is able to move about, he should take Epsom salt baths twice weekly. The procedure for taking this bath has been explained in the appendix. He should also take breathing and other exercises daily, along with daily friction and sponge as explained in the appendix. The consumption of alcoholic beverages and smoking should be completely given up.

Liberal use of fruits and vegetables has been found beneficial in the prevention and treatment of stroke. Research carried out more than a decade ago, indicated that consuming fruits and vegetables prevented strokes and reduced the damage if they occurred. British scientists at Cambridge University discovered that older persons who consumed large quantities of fresh green vegetables and fresh fruits were less likely to die of strokes. A Norwegian study found that men who consumed liberal amounts of vegetables had a 45 per cent lower risk of stroke. It also found that women who consumed lots of fruits were one-third less likely to have a stroke.

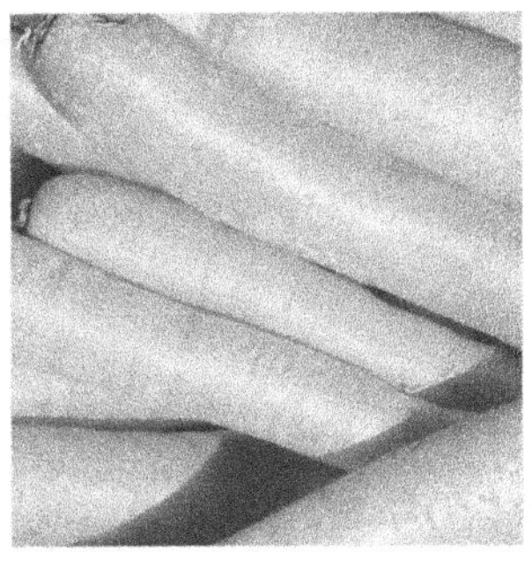

Carrots have been found very valuable in stroke. A recent Harvard study has shown that eating carrots five times a week or more can reduce the risk of stroke drastically by two-thirds, compared with eating carrots only once a month or less. This conclusion was reached after observing nearly 90,000 women nurses for eight years.

Spinach is another vegetable found valuable in the prevention and treatment of stroke. The protection seems to come partly from beta carotene in carrots and spinach. A previous Harvard study found that eating the extra beta carotene in about one and a half carrots, which equals 200 g of mashed sweet potatoes or 170 g spinach (weighed raw and then cooked) every day saved 40 per cent off stroke rates. The drop was evident in those who ate 15-20 mg of beta carotene daily compared to those who ate only 6 mg. The antistroke activity in carrots, spinach and other carotene-rich vegetables seems to emanate from their antioxidant properties.

Another new research study has shown that lots of beta carotene and other Vitamin A in the blood stream can prevent death in case stroke occurs. This conclusion has been reached by

Belgian researchers at the University of Brussels, who analysed the blood of 80 patients within 24 hours after they had suffered strokes. When the brain is deprived of oxygen, as in a stroke, cells begin to malfunction, leading to a series of events culminating in oxidative damage to nerve cells, but if there is lot of Vitamin A in the blood, it appears to interfere at many different stages of events, reducing brain damage and chances of death.

Other foods rich in beta carotene, besides carrots, are dark green leafy vegetables and orange coloured vegetables and fruits such as spinach, pumpkin, sweet potatoes, tomatoes, oranges, papayas, mangoes and melon.

Potassium is another potent antidote against strokes. Eating just one extra serving of potassium-rich food every day, may reduce the risk of stroke by 40 per cent. Researchers have discovered this by analysing the diets of a group of 859 men and women over the age 50 years, living in Southern California.

It was remarkable that none of the persons who took substantial quantities of potassium died of a stroke, but those who regularly consumed very little potassium had much higher fatal stroke rates than all the others. Among those who took least potassium, stroke deaths shot up 2.6 times in men and 4.8 times in women. Further, the more potassium-rich foods the subjects ate, generally the fewer strokes they had. The researchers concluded that with every extra daily 400 mg of potassium in food, the odds of a fatal stroke dropped by 40 per cent. This critical margin of 400 mg of potassium is so modest that one can obtain it in a single piece of most fruits and vegetables and a glass of milk.

Fresh air and outdoor exercise, as far as possible, correct diet along the lines outlined above, and clean wholesome living will prevent occurrence of further strokes. All undue nervous excitement, needless worry and excessive strain must be avoided.

CHAPTER 14

Parkinson's Disease

Parkinson's disease, also known as paralysis against or shaking palsy, is a serious chronic disease of the nervous system. It is characterised by stiffness of muscles and a continual tremor or shake. It is a disease of the extrapyramidal system.

Parkinson's disease is widely prevalent in old age and is largely regarded as a disease of the elderly. It affects one to two per cent of those aged 60 years or over. The incidence rises further with advancing age. An epidemological study by Godwin and Austen in 1982 has shown that 58 per cent sufferers in Britain are aged 70 or more.

Symptoms

The description of the disease originally given by Dr. James Parkinson of Shoreditch in 1817 is as follows: 'Involuntary tremulous motion, with lessened muscular power, in parts not in action and even when supported, with a propensity to bend the trunk forwards, and to pass from a walking to a running pace, the senses and intellect being uninjured.' The patient shows a combination of tremors of the limbs and muscular stiffness. These tremors are more noticeable when the patient is at rest, and tend to disappear when he attempts to move or when he is asleep. The tremors are more pronounced, when he is excited or fatigued.

Older patients occasionally exhibit involuntary rapid jerking movement of their arms and legs. In a less extreme form the condition presents as purposeless mastication and lip smacking movements. The condition is embarrassing both to the patient and his relatives, but is not associated with mental impairment and rarely causes severe incapacity.

Later, there may be impairment of speech, and the patient may complain of cramping pains in the back because of muscle spasm. His mind usually remains clear, and his other sensations are normal. In many cases, the patient may have only a mild form of Parkinson's disease and continue this way for many years before any serious symptoms develop. In severe and advanced cases, however, the patient is not able to move, and presents a distressing spectacle, for his mind may be uninjured while he cannot speak or write.

Causes

Parkinson's disease may follow severe attacks of encephalitis or some type of poisoning, such as carbon monoxide. In older patients, this type of palsy may be due to hardening of the arteries in certain vessels leading to the brain. In most cases, however, the disease begins to show itself in later middle age, and is considered to be a consequence of 'degeneration,' particularly in the basal ganglia.

Parkinson's disease may also result from deficiency of antioxidant Vitamin E earlier in life. According to Dr. Lawrence Golbe, MD, a neurologist at the University of Medicine and Dentistry of New Jersey, too little Vitamin E foods earlier in life may somehow leave the brain vulnerable to the onset of Parkinson's disease years later. In most cases of Parkinson's disease, the cause is unknown.

Treatment

Diet plays an important role in the treatment of this disease. To begin with, the patient should resort to a short juice fast for

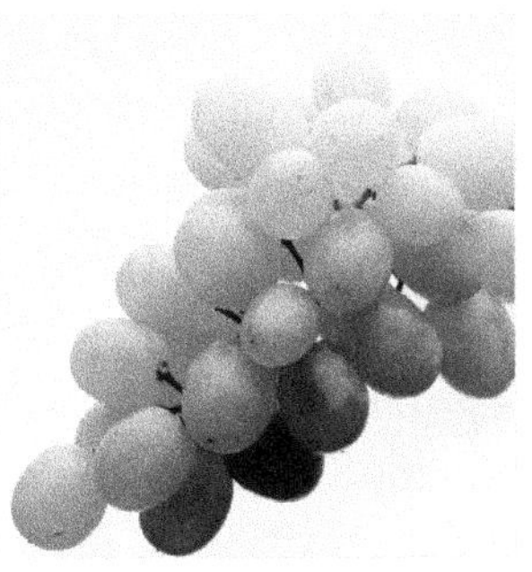

five days. In this regimen, he should take a glass of fresh fruit or vegetable juice, diluted with water on 50:50 basis, every two hours from 8 a.m. to 8 p.m. Fruits and vegetables which may be used for juicing are apple, pineapple, grapes, orange, tomato, carrot, cabbage and spinach. A warm water enema should be used daily to cleanse the bowels during the period of fasting.

After the short juice fast, the patient may adopt an all-fruit diet for further 5 days. During this period, he should take three meals a day of fresh juicy fruits, such as apple, pear, peach, papaya, grapes, orange and pineapple, at five-hourly intervals. Thereafter, he may gradually adopt a well-balanced lacto-vegetarian diet. The emphasis should be on raw seeds, nuts and grains, plenty of sprouts, raw milk, preferably goat's milk, and raw fruits and vegetables. Green leafy vegetables and yellow turnips are especially beneficial. Sesame seeds and sesame seed butter can be taken with beneficial results. In general, a low-protein diet of raw, organically grown foods is best for the patient with Parkinson's disease.

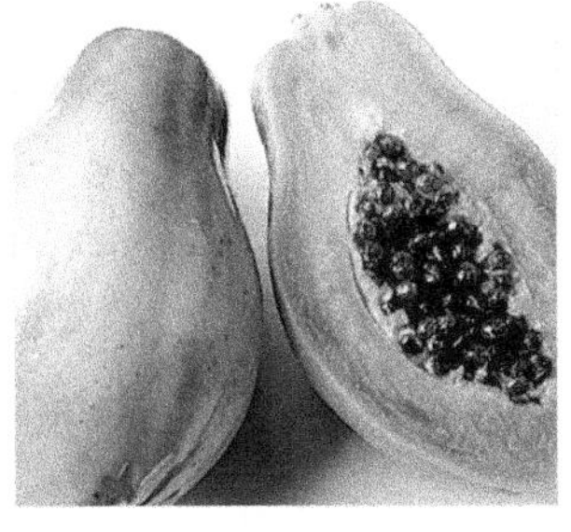

The patient should avoid tea, coffee, chocolate, salt, spices, condiments, pickles, fresh foods, white flour and white sugar and all processed, tinned, canned and frozen foods. The short juice fast followed by an all-fruit diet should be repeated at monthly intervals till conditions improves.

Use of Vitamin E in high doses is considered beneficial on the treatment of Parkinson's disease. There is preliminary evidence to suggest that massive doses of Vitamin E, say, 800 to 3,000 international units daily, may slow down the progress of the disease. Extensive studies about the efficacy of the Vitamin E therapy for Parkinson's disease are, however, still being carried out.

Everything possible should be done to help the patient to maintain a cheerful mental outlook. He should remain as active as possible and lead a quiet life. Hot moist packs may be applied to the stiffened muscles which should also be gently massaged. The daily warm bath is useful. Fresh air and light exercise, especially walking, are essential to the treatment of Parkinson's disease.

CHAPTER 15

Insomnia

The term insomnia literally denotes a complete lack of sleep. It is, however, used to indicate a relative inability to sleep that consists of difficulty in falling asleep, difficulty staying asleep, early final awakening or combination of these complaints. Insomnia deprives the person of mental rest and thereby interferes with his activities in the daytime. It constitutes a severe health hazard when it becomes a habit.

Insomnia has assumed alarming proportions of late, especially among the upper classes in the urban set-up. Numerous surveys have been conducted about sleep disturbance in the general population. These surveys have revealed a close relationship between advancing age and disturbed sleep. This is also established by the recent drug surveys indicating disproportionately large number of prescriptions for sleep written by physicians for patients over the age of 60 years.

Insomnia is common among the elderly for a variety of reasons. The sleep of the elderly is often punctuated by brief periods of wakefulness during the night. In such cases, it is the quality rather than the quantity which is most affected. With age, there is a gradual reduction of periods of deep sleep. The older persons, therefore, gets roused earlier. Sleep requirements also diminish with ageing. From nine hours of sleep per night at the age of 12, the average sleep needs decrease to eight hours at the age of 20, seven hours at 40, six and a half hours at 60 and six hours at 80. There also appears to be a tendency among the elderly individuals to advance their usual bedtime with age and to arise at an earlier hour.

Symptoms

The signs of pathological insomnia are dramatic changes in the duration and quality of sleep, persistent changes in sleep patterns, lapses of memory and lack of concentration during the day. Other symptoms are emotional instability, loss of co-ordination, confusion and a lingering feeling of indifference.

Causes

The most common cause of sleeplessness is mental tension brought about by anxiety, worries, overwork and overexcitement. Suppressed feelings of resentment, anger and bitterness may also cause insomnia. Constipation, dyspepsia, overeating at night, excessive intake of tea or coffee and going to bed hungry are among the other causes. Smoking is another unsuspected cause of insomnia as it irritates the nervous system. Often, worrying about falling asleep is enough to keep one awake.

There is consensus among sleep specialists that physical conditions, drugs and alcohol are collectively more significant factors in causing sleeplessness among older persons than major psychiatric conditions. This can be attributed to the fact that neurotic elderly rarely come to the attention of sleep specialists and hardly anything is known about their sleep complaints.

Treatment

Sleeping pills are not remedy for sleeplessness. They are habit forming and become less effective when taken continuously. They lower the I. Q. and dull the brain. To overcome the problem, the older person should adhere to a regular sleeping schedule, going to bed at a fixed time each night and getting up at a fixed time each morning. Early to bed and early to rise is a good rule. Two hours of sleep before midnight are more beneficial than four hours after.

Research has shown that people with chronic insomnia almost invariably have marked deficiencies of such key nutrients as B complex vitamins, and Vitamin C and D as also calcium, magnesium, manganese, potassium and zinc. The sleep mechanism is unable to function efficiently unless each of these nutrients is present in adequate amounts in the diet.

A balanced diet with simple modification in the eating pattern will go a long way in the treatment of insomnia. Such a diet should exclude white flour products, sugar and its products, tea, coffee, chocolate, cola drinks, alcohol, fatty foods, fried foods, foods containing additives, excessive use of salt and strong condiments.

In the modified eating pattern, breakfast should consist of fresh and dried fruits, seeds and milk or yogurt. Of the two main meals, one should consist of a large mixed salad of raw vegetables and the other should be protein based. A cup of milk sweetened with honey at bedtime is helpful as the amino-acid tryptophan contained in milk induces sleep.

Certain home remedies have been found beneficial in the treatment of insomnia. One of the most effective of these remedies is the use of lettuce (salad-ka-patta). The juice of this plant has been likened in effect to the sedative action of opium without the accompanying excitement. The seeds of lettuce in decoction form are also useful in insomnia.

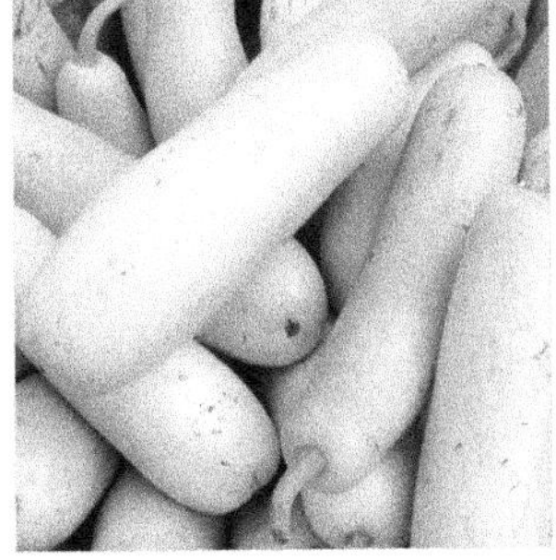

The mixture of bottle gourd (lauki) juice and sesame oil acts as an effective medicine for insomnia. It should be massaged over scalp every night. The cooked leaves of bottle gourd taken as a vegetable are also beneficial in the treatment of this disease.

A tea made from aniseed (saunf) is valuable in sleeplessness. This tea is prepared by boiling about 375 ml. of water in a vessel and adding a teaspoon of aniseed. The water should be covered with a lid and allowed to simmer for 15 minutes. It should then be strained and drunk hot or warm. The tea may be sweetened with honey and hot milk may also be added to it. This tea should be taken after meals or before going to bed.

Another effective remedy for insomnia is the use of honey. It has hypnotic action in bringing sound sleep. It should be taken with water, before going to bed, in doses of two teaspoons in a cup of water. People generally fall asleep after taking honey.

Controlled breathing is a great help in inducing sleep. The method is to lie on your side in bed and then take three deep breaths expanding the abdomen completely. Then hold your breath as long as you can. Next, take three more breaths and repeat the breath-holding. While you hold breath, carbon dioxide accumulates in the body and induces natural sleep.

Regular active exercise during the day and mild exercise at bedtime enhances the quantity and the quality of sleep. Exercise stimulates the elimination of lactic acid from the body which co-relates with stress and muscular tension. Regular exercise also produces hormonal changes which are beneficial to the body and to the sleep pattern. Walking, jogging, swimming are all ideal exercises.

Yoga helps a majority of cases of insomnia in the elderly. It helps tone up the glandular, respiratory and nervous systems. It also gives physical and mental relaxation as a safety value for one's disturbing problems. The yogasanas effective for insomnia patients are sarvangasana, uttanasana, viparitakarni and shavasana.

Hydrotherapy is also effective in the treatment of insomnia. Application of hot packs to the spine before retiring, hot fomentation to the spine, hot foot bath at bedtime are all time-tested methods. Prolonged neutral immersion bath (92° to 96° F) at bed time, when one's nerves are usually irritable, is also an effective measure. The procedure for taking this bath has been explained in the appendix.

Along with the various measures for the treatment of insomnia, the patient should make all efforts to eliminate as many stress factors as possible. The steps in this direction should include regular practices of any relaxation method or meditation technique, cultivating the art of doing things slowly, particularly activities like eating, walking and talking, cultivating a creative hobby and spending some time daily on this, avoiding working against unrealistic targets and completing one's task before starting another.

CHAPTER 16

Headaches

Headaches affect almost everyone at some time or the other. Most headaches are functional, caused by temporary upsets and are not related to any organic changes in the brain. A headache is often nature's warning that something is wrong somewhere in the body. The actual pain, however, arises from irritation to nerve endings in the shoulder, neck and scalp muscles and also in the smooth muscles encircling the blood vessels which serve these areas.

Causes

The most common cause of headache is allergy, especially allergy to certain foods. According to Dr. David W. Buchholz, M.D., Director of the neurological Consultation clinic at Johns Hopkins University Hospital, the most common food suspects which trigger headaches are chocolate, strong cheese, caffeine in coffee, tea and cola, yoghurt, processed, cured and preserved meats, alcoholic drinks, citrus fruits such as oranges, grapefruit, lemons, lime and pineapples and their juices, other fruits like bananas, raisins, red plums, canned figs, and avocados and certain vegetables like broad beans, peas and onions. Sneezing and diarrhoea are further indications of an allergy.

Another important cause of headaches is intense emotion. Many people who outwardly appear to have a pleasant disposition may actually be simmering about a job, or may bear resentment towards a person or something. This hidden hostility may manifest itself as headache. It is important, therefore, that negative feelings should not be bottled up, but should find some safe means of expression.

Migraine can cause severe headache, generally on one side of the head. It is also known as sick headache because nausea and vomitting occasionally accompany the excruciating pain which lasts for as long as three days. Migraine usually gives warning before it strikes: black spots or a brilliant zig-zag line appear before the eyes or the patient has blurring of vision or has part of his vision blanked out. When headache occurs, the patients may feel tingling, numbness, or weakness in an arm or leg. Other causes of headache are eye strain, high blood pressure, infection, low blood sugar, nutritional deficiency, tension and the presence of poisons and toxins in the body.

Headache is less common in old age than in younger age groups. Although it is quite frequent in the elderly depressed and psychoneurotic patients, the tension headache, so often complained of by younger anxious patients, is unusual in the elderly, Migraine may persist into old age, but it is usually less troublesome than before. It may completely disappear in some former sufferers. Migraine rarely makes its first appearance in old age.

Perhaps the most common cause of headache in an elderly person is cervical spondylitis. The pain mainly occurs in the hindmost bone of the skull but may radiate forwards to the vertex. The movements of the neck are usually grossly limited and rotation of the neck aggravates the pain.

Treatment

Taking an aspirin or a tranquiliser may provide temporary relief, but it does not remove the cause, moreover, the frequent use of pain-relievers causes nervous debility, weakens the heart and brings in other complications.

The best remedy to prevent headaches is to build up physical resistance through proper nutrition, exercise and constructive thinking. As a first step, the patient should undertake short juice fast. During this period, fresh fruit and vegetable juices, diluted with water on 50:50 basis, may be taken six times daily. By taking the load off the digestion, the patient will at once save nervous energy which can be utilised for more important purposes. The blood and lymph will also be relieved of a great burden. After a short juice fast, the diet should be fixed in such a way as to put the least possible strain on the digestion. Breakfast should consist of fruits, both fresh and dried. Lunch should consist largely of protein foods. Starchy foods such as whole wheat bread, cereals, rice, or potatoes should be taken at dinner along with raw salads. Spices, tomatoes, sour buttermilk and oily foodstuffs should be avoided.

Diet factor is of utmost importance in treating headaches. Dr. David W. Buchholz believes that the single easiest headache-provoking factor one can control is the diet. Thus, avoiding food culprits can be crucial in preventing headaches. He feels that headaches can be prevented by identifying and avoiding foods that trigger headache. His advice is to avoid for one month all foods most likely to trigger headaches and also caffeine-containing medications and painkillers. If the headaches subside or disappear, one can then experiment by adding back a food item one at a time every three days or once a week. If a headache occurs, one will then know the food which is a headache trigger and should avoid it. Dr. Buchholz cautions that it may take 24 hours after consuming a food for a headache to show up. After one determines which foods trigger headaches, one can avoid them. However, he recommends not adding caffeine back into the diet, if one has frequent headaches.

Home Remedies

Certain home remedies have been found beneficial in the

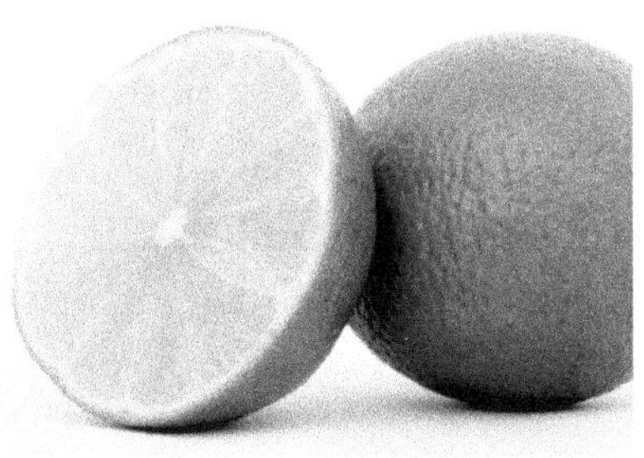

treatment of various types of headaches. Lemon (bara nimbu) is valuable in bilious headache. The juice of three or four slices of this fruit should be squeezed in a cup of water and drunk by the patient for treating this condition. The crust of lemon, which is generally thrown away, has been found useful in headaches caused by heat. Lemon crusts should be pounded into a fine paste in a mortar and applied as plaster on the forehead. It will give relief. Applying yellow rind of a lemon, newly pared off, to each temple will also give relief.

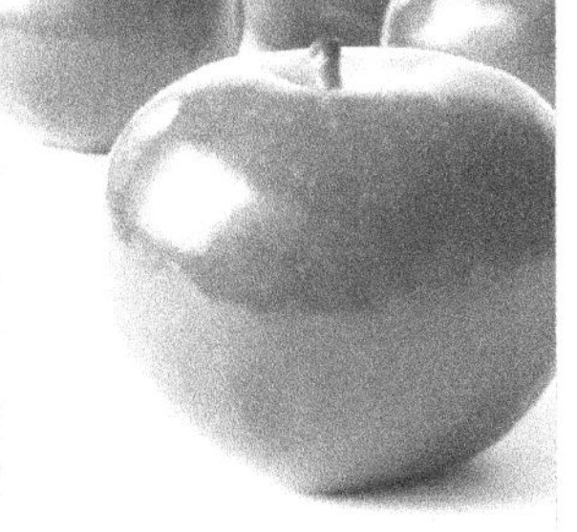

Apples (seb) are valuable in all types of headaches. A ripe apple, after removing the upper rind and the inner hard portion, should be taken with a little salt every morning. This should be continued for about a week.

The flowers of henna (mehndi) have been found valuable in headaches caused by hot sun. A plaster of the flowers should be prepared by rubbing them in vinegar and applied over the forehead. It will soon give relief. Cinnamon (dalchini) is useful in headaches caused by exposure to cold air. A fine paste of this spice should be prepared by mixing it with water and it should be applied over the temples and forehead to obtain relief.

Certain water applications help relieve headaches. Copious drinking of water can help as do the cleansing enema with water temperature at 98.60° F, the hot foot bath, a cold throat pack, frequent applications of towels wrung out from very hot water to the back of the neck, a cold compress at 40° to 60° F applied to the head and face or an alternate spinal compress. Hot fomentations over the abdominal region just before retiring relieve headaches due to stomach and liver upsets.

Yogic kriyas like jalneti and kunjal, pranayamas like anulome-viloma, shitali and sitkari and asanas such as uttanpadasana, sarvangasana, paschimottanasana, halasana and shavasana are useful in the treatment of headaches.

CHAPTER 17

Cervical Spondylosis

Cervical spondylosis is a degenerative disease of cervical region of the spine and is commonly prevalent in old age. It results from degeneration of intervertebral disc and consequent pressure on the cervical nerve roots or cervical spinal cord. It is an arthritic process involving the vertebra, and is often associated with osteoarthritis in the rest of the skeleton.

The spine is a vital part of the back which is known as life bone of the body. The back is a complex structure of muscles, bones and elastic tissues. The spine is made of 24 blocks of bone piled one on top of the other. Sandwiched between these bony blocks are cushions of the cartilage and elastic tissues, called intervertebral discs. The vertebral discs act as shock absorbers for the back. Mobility would be impossible without these discs. Cervical spondylosis occurs due to the narrowing of the space between the cervical vertebra resulting in the compression of the nerves.

Symptoms

The main symptom of cervical spondylosis is nagging and severe pain. The pain may spread over to both sides of shoulders, back side of neck, the collar bone and head. In some cases, pain may occur in both the arm and fingers. Some people may also get pain in the chest and throat. Another important symptom of this disease is stiffness, which may be acute or chronic. It may lead to the restricted movements, which may be partial or complete or movement may be limited. Other symptoms of cervical spondylosis are numbness and tingling or complete loss of sensation on the affected side, headache and giddiness. Occasionally, there may be weakness of the muscles, of the arm or hand. Diagnosis can be confirmed by an x-ray of the spine.

Causes

The main causes of cervical spondylosis are injury, faulty posture, incorrect nutrition resulting from dietic errors, psychological strain leading to the muscle spasm and lack of exercise. The disease may follow an injury, sustained many years ago, particularly neck injury, caused by an accident. Other causes include stress and strain resulting from sitting for a long time, improper lifting of weights and emotional problems which may cause painful muscle cramping.

Poor posture results from soft chairs and coaches, which facilitate slouching and sitting incorrectly. Sleeping on too soft a mattress which results in an improper back and neck posture, can cause tension, headaches and pain in the upper and lower back. Lack of exercise is another important cause of spondylosis. Modern conveniences have made office work easier. When muscles are not exercised and remain weak, the chances of injury to them is increased manifold.

Treatment

Drugs prescribed to relieve pain or relax muscles in cervical spondylosis do not cure the disease. These can become habit forming and may actually perpetuate the condition in case of excessive intake.

Certain safety measures, especially for people in sedentary occupations, are necessary to relieve and prevent spondylosis. The most important of these is exercise which improves the supply of nutrients to spinal discs, thereby delaying the process of deterioration that comes with age and eventually affects everybody. Safe exercises include walking, swimming and bicycling. The latter should be done keeping the back upright.

Other exercises found beneficial in the treatment of cervical spondylosis are joint movements like folding and unfolding of fingers, moving the wrists up and down, rotating them in both clockwise and anti-clockwise direction, folding and unfolding of the forearms and rotating the shoulder clockwise and anti-clockwise; head and neck exercises like moving the neck up and down, moving to the sides, rotating the neck clockwise and anti-clockwise and nodding the neck from one shoulder to another; and shoulder exercises like lifting the shoulders up and down, moving the shoulder in clockwise and in anti-clockwise directions. All these exercises should be undertaken three times daily.

Those with sedentary occupations should take a break to stand up every hour. Soft-cushioned seats should be avoided and position should be changed as often as possible. Elderly persons with spondylosis should sleep on a firm mattress on their sides with knees bent at right angles to the torso. They should use thin pillows or avoid it altogether, if possible. They should take care never to bend from the waist down to lift any object, but instead should squat close to the object, bending the knees but keeping the back straight and then stand up slowly.

The diet of elderly persons suffering from spondylosis should consist of salad of raw vegetables such as tomato, carrot, cabbage, cucumber, radish, lettuce and at least two steamed or lightly-cooked vegetables such as cauliflower, cabbage, carrot, spinach and plenty of fruits. The patients

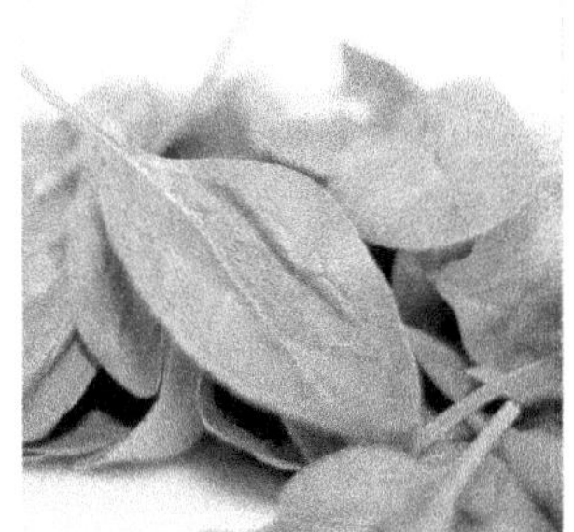

should have four meals daily. They may take fruits and milk for breakfast, steamed vegetables and whole wheat chapattis during lunch, fresh fruit or fruit juice in the evening and a bowl of raw salad and sprouts during dinner.

The patient should avoid fatty, spicy and fried foods, sour curd, sweets, sugar, condiments as well as tea and coffee.

Those who smoke and take tobacco in any form should give up completely.

Proteins and Vitamin C are necessary for the development of a healthy bone metrix. Vitamin D, calcium, phosphorous and the essential trace minerals are essential for healthy bones. Foods that have been processed for storage to avoid spoiling have few nutrients and should be eliminated from the diet.

Certain food remedies have been found beneficial in the treatment of spondylosis. The most important of these is the use of garlic. Two or three capsules of this vegetable should be taken daily in the morning. It will give good results. An oil prepared from garlic and rubbed on the affected part will give great relief. This oil is prepared by frying 10 cloves of garlic in 60 gms of oil in a frying pan. They should be fried slowly till they are brown. After it is cooled, it should be applied vigorously on the affected part and allowed to remain there for three hours. The patient may thereafter have a warm bath. This treatment should be continued for at least 15 days.

Relief from pain can be obtained by taking lemon juice mixed with common salt twice or thrice daily. A piece of the chebulic myrobalan (harad or haritaki) taken after principal meals also gives quick relief.

Other measures found valuable in cervical spondylosis are mild oil massage to the neck, shoulders and hands, hot fomentation for five to 10 minutes twice a day or five to 10 minutes of exposure to the Infra red rays. Yogic asanas which are beneficial in the treatment of spondylosis are bhujangasana, shalabhasana, vakrasana, uttanpadasana and shavasana.

CHAPTER 18

Falls

Falls is a common and most frightening nervous disorder in advanced old age. A fall occurs when the vertical line which passes through the centre of the mass of the human body comes to lie beyond the support base and correction does not take place in time.

There are two types of falls in the elderly. The young old person falls occasionally because he unwisely indulges in activities involving large and rapid displacements of which he was once capable, but which now exceeds his capacity. In the second type, the older people who suffer from multiple disabilities, fall frequently due to the sharp decline in the efficiency of balance mechanism.

Most falls are trivial and they do not result in injury. It is estimated that nearly 80 per cent of falls do not result in injury. In other cases, injuries may result depending on the intensity and rapidity of the fall. Older people most likely to suffer injury are those who are moving rapidly at the time of the fall.

Causes

Falls may be caused by a variety of factors. The elderly people with recurrent falls usually have a continuing cause. Some people lose consciousness before or after the fall. Momentary loss of consciousness may result from epilepsy and circulatory disturbances. Temporary loss of consciousness in old age is usually caused by a temporary disturbance of cerebral circulation resulting from a fall in cardiac output or an error in blood distribution.

Falls may also be caused by normal initiated displacement or excessive initiated displacement. The former consists of activities of daily living like getting out of bed, rising from a chair, walking, dressing and sitting down. The latter takes place when ordinary activities are conducted in haste or without preparation or when actions are undertaken without due thoughts. Excessive use of drugs can also lead to instability, resulting in falls. Most of the old people habitually take too many drugs for treating various ailments, including sedatives and tranquillisers, and this can affect the slowing in central conduction of the nervous system, causing instability.

Most falls occur while walking. These falls may result from neurological diseases like strokes, weakness of the legs and failure to raise the feet, multiple sclerosis and Parkinson's disease. These diseases affect rhythmicity and regularity of stepping, thereby endangering stability.

Treatment

All efforts should be made to improve the performance of the patient. The most important step in this direction is to create confidence in the patient's own ability to remain upright throughout his daily activities. Other steps in this direction include provision of well-fitting shoes with low heels to the patient and improvements in his environment like appropriate floor surface and floor coverings, proper arrangement of furniture, adequate lighting and correct height of chairs and beds. This is essential as some old people are used to walking frames or to clutching on to furniture as they move around the house. Those patients who have recently developed the tendency to fall and are able to maintain balance, should be discouraged from using walking frames as they alter the body postures and the pattern of walking.

Proper training of the patient is also an important factor in treating the condition. They should be encouraged to walk with confidence and supported, if necessary, by a hand held lightly in front of them. The patient's training should aim at increasing his speed of walking as the more rapidly he walks, within limit, the safer he appears to be. While climbing stairs, the patient should take the support of the railing with one hand and should concentrate on placing the feet carefully and firmly on the steps. He should be encouraged to practise transfers from bed to chair, from chair to toilet and so on. Those who are at a risk of falling and who have shown their inability to rise without assistance, should be taught the proper technique to get up, which is to turn on to the side and to bend up one knee. From this position they should be able to roll on to that knee and to bring up the second knee until they are kneeling. They may then be able to crawl or to reach out for a nearby chair and gradually get up with its support.

The patient with a tendency to fall should be given optimum nutrition, well-assimilated with all the vitamins and other nutrients. The emphasis should be on whole grains, particularly whole wheat, brown rice, raw and sprouted seeds, milk, especially in soured form and home-made cottage cheese.

In this regimen, the breakfast may consist of fresh fruits, handful of raw nuts or a couple of tablespoons of sunflower and pumpkin seeds. Steamed vegetables, whole wheat chapattis and a glass of buttermilk may be taken for lunch. The dinner may comprise a large bowl of fresh, green, vegetable salad, fresh home-made cottage cheese, fresh butter and a glass of buttermilk.

In severe cases, the patients should be put on a short juice fast for four or five days before being given the optimum diet. Carrot, beet, citrus fruits, apple and pineapple may be used for juices.

All vitamins of the B group have proved beneficial in the prevention and treatment of nervous disorders. The tendency to recurrent falls can be helped by liberal intake of Vitamin B1, B2, B6, B12 and pantothenic acid which should be given together.

The patient should avoid white bread, white sugar, refined cereals, meat, fish, tinned foods, tea, coffee and condiments which are at the root of the trouble, by continuously flooding the tissues with acid impurities.

Soyabean milk is considered beneficial in the treatment of nervous disorders. A cupful of soyabean milk mixed with a teaspoonful of honey should be taken every night in this condition. It tones up the nervous system due to its rich concentration of lecithin, Vitamin B1 and glutanic acid.

The patient should be given two or three hot epsom-salt baths weekly. He should remain in the bath for 25 to 30 minutes. The procedure for taking this bath has been given in the appendix. The patient should undertake walking and other moderate exercises.

SECTION III

LOW VISION

CHAPTER 19

Low Vision

Impairment of vision occurs almost universally in later life. This seems to be caused by biological factors. It is usually accepted as a sign of ageing process. It is quite unusual to come across an elderly person with perfect vision at all distances in both eyes. Those who perform all visual tasks normally without glasses generally have some degree of myopia in one eye only and have a normal refraction in the other.

There is gradual deterioration in vision in old age. Deterioration is more likely to be continuous after the age of 65 years. The most common refractive problem in the elderly is long-sightedness. Old people often find that their vision is seriously impaired when there is poor light. They may, however, have good vision when the light is adequate.

The most important reason for impairment of vision in old age is degenerative conditions of the retina. There are also changes in the pupil which commonly affect visual performance. It changes in respect of both, size and agility. There is a decrease in its diameter which reduces the amount of light reaching the retina. Senile muscular degeneration may lead to a serious impairment of central vision but may not affect peripheral vision, so that elderly persons do not become totally blind.

Causes

The main causes of low vision which is not associated with degenerative changes, are mental strain, wrong feeding and improper blood and nerve supply. Dr. W. H. Bates, the founder of revolutionary methods of eye treatment, considers mental strain to be the cause of all defects of vision, which puts corresponding physical strain on the eyes, their muscles and nerves. In his opinion, the lesser defects are mainly due to mental strain owing to overwork, fear, anxiety, etc. In pursuance of this theory. Dr. Bates has concentrated his efforts on methods of treatment which will remove the condition of mental strain.

The eye is a part of the body and as such must share in any condition affecting the system. Most of the disease affecting the eyes are symptoms of a general toxemic condition of the body due mainly to ingestion of excessive starch, sugar and protein. The muscles and blood vessels surrounding the eyes share in the clogging process taking place over the body due to improper metabolism caused by an imbalanced and too concentrated diet.

The eyes need to be properly supplied with blood and nerve force for proper vision. Any factor capable of interfering either with the blood-vessels or with the nerves of the eyes could cause defective vision. The muscles covering the upper portion of the spine at the back of the neck are the main seat of mechanical interference with the blood and nerve supply to the eyes.

Treatment

The stained and contracted muscles surrounding the eyes can be loosened by certain eye and neck exercises. These exercises are as follows:

Eye exercises

(i) Keep your head still and relaxed. Gently move the eyes up and down six times. Repeat the same movement twice or thrice at two seconds intervals. The eyes should move slowly and regularly as far down as possible and then as far up as possible.

(ii) Move the eyes from side to side as far as possible, without any force or effort six times. Repeat two or three times.

(iii) Hold the index finger of your right hand about eight inches in front of the eyes, then look from the finger to any other large object ten or more feet away — the door or window will do. Look from one to the other ten times. Do this exercise fairly rapidly.

(iv) Move the eyes up gently and slowly in a circle, then move them low in the reverse direction. Do this four times in all. Rest for a second and repeat the movements two or three times, using minimum effort. All eye muscle exercises should be performed while seated in a comfortable position.

Neck exercises: Rotate the neck (a) in circles and semicircles, (b) move the shoulders clockwise and anti-clockwise briskly, drawing them up as far as possible several times, (c) allow the head to drop forward and backward as far as possible, (d) turn the head to the right and left as far as possible several times. These exercises help to loosen up contracted neck muscles which may restrict blood supply to the head.

Other measures: Other measures which can help defective vision are as follows:

Sun gazing: Sit on a bench facing the sun with your eyes closed and gently sway sideways several times for 18 minutes. Open the eyes and blink about 10 times at the sun and look at some greenery. This helps shortsight and is good for inflammed eyes.

Splashing: Splash plain, cold water several times on closed eyes. Rub the closed lids briskly for a minute with a clean towel. This cools the eyes and boosts blood supply.

Palming: Sit comfortably in an armchair or on a settee and relax with your eyes closed. Cover your eyes with your palms, right palm over the right eye and the left over the left eye. Do not, however, press down on the eyes. With your eyes completely covered in this manner, allow your elbows to drop to your knees, which would be fairly close together. With your eyes closed thus, try to imagine blackness, which grows blacker and blacker. Palming reduces strain and relaxes the eyes and its surrounding tissues.

Swinging: Stand with your feet 12 inches apart, hands held loosely at the sides; the whole body and mind relaxed. Gently sway your body from side to side, slowly, steadily with the heels rising alternatively but not the rest of the foot. Imagine you are the pendulum of a clock, and move just as slowly. Swinging should be done in front of a window or a picture. You will see the object moving in the opposite direction of your swing. This must be noted and encouraged. When you face one end of the window or object, blink once. This exercise has a very beneficial effect upon the eyes and nervous system.

Diet

Natural, uncooked foods are the best diet. These include fresh fruits such as oranges, apples, grapes, peaches, plums, cherries; green vegetables like lettuce, cabbage, spinach, turnip tops, root vegetables like potatoes, turnips, carrot, onions and beetroots; nuts, dried fruits and dairy products.

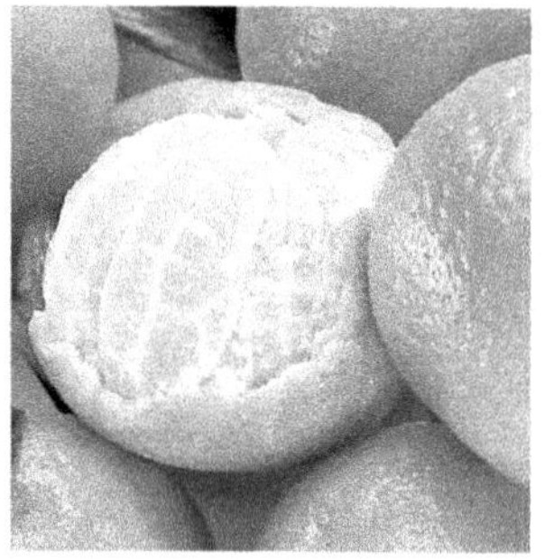

Cereals are also necessary, but they should be consumed sparingly. Genuine wholemeal bread is the best and most suitable. Cakes, pastries, white sugar, white bread, tea, coffee, etc., together with meat, fish, or eggs, play havoc with the digestion and the body.

The value of Vitamin A for improving vision must be stressed. The intake of sufficient quantities of this vitamin is essential as a safeguard against or treatment of defective vision or eye disease of any kind. The best sources of this vitamin are codliver oil, raw spinach, turnip tops, cream, cheese, butter, egg yolk, tomatoes, lettuce, carrot, cabbage, soya beans, green peas, fresh milk, oranges and dates.

Yogic Exercises

In Yoga, four exercises have been prescribed for strengthening weak eye muscles, relieving eye strain and curing of eye disease. They are known as "Trataka" which in Sanskrit means "Winkless gaze at a particular point", or looking at an object with awareness. The four tratakas are: Dakshinayjatru trataka in which, with face forwards, the eyes are fixed on the tip of the right shoulder; Vamajatru trataka, in which the eyes are fixed on the tip of the left shoulder; Namikagra trataka, in which the eyes are focussed on the tip of the nose, and Bhrumadhya trataka, in which the eyes are focussed on the space between the eyebrows. These exercises should be practised from a meditative position like padmasana or vajrasana. The gaze should be maintained for as long as you are comfortable, gradually increasing the period from 10 to 20 and then to 30 seconds. The eyes should be closed and rested after each exercise. Persons with acute myopia should perform the tratakas with their eyes closed.

Certain yoga asanas such as bhujangasana, shalabhasana, yogamudra, paschimottanasana and kriyas like jalneti are also beneficial for the eyes.

CHAPTER 20

Cataract

Cataract is one of the most common eye diseases. The term actually means a waterfall and refers to the opacity of the crystalline lens of the eye on the assumption that the condition is caused by the humour of the brain falling over the pupil.

The crystalline lens, through which light travels into the interior of the eye, is situated just behind the iris, or coloured portion of the eye. In cataract, this lens becomes opaque, thus seriously hampering the entrance of light into the eye. Blindness ensues when no light rays can permeate the opacity of the lens.

Cataract is almost unavoidable in old age. All of us develop some degree of opacity in the lens after 50 years of age. This obscures vision and leads to difficulties in focusing on near objects as the years go by. However, only some people develop a greater degree of opacity to require surgery. The progress of the conditions is not continuous but intermittent in many cases and also not symmetrical between eyes. Surgical removal of the cataract is necessary once it gets matured.

During the time the cataract progresses towards maturity, the vision decreases considerably. It is therefore important that elderly persons get their vision checked regularly and change their glasses accordingly. Or else they may tend to fall more frequently and may even break their bones. This will cause emotional stress in the patient and in the family members as well.

Symptoms

The first sign of cataract is blurred vision. The patient finds it difficult to see things in focus. As the cataract progresses, the patient may get double vision or spots or both. There is gradual increase in blindness. At first, vision in twilight may be better than in full daylight since light is admitted round the more widely-dilated pupil in the dark. In the advance stage, objects and persons may appear merely blobs of light. In the final stage, there is a grayish white discoloration in the pupil.

Causes

Cataract is often found in association with other defects of the eye. There are four factors which contribute to the loss of transparency of the lens. These are stagnation of the fluid current in the lens due to blood condition; deterioration in the nutrition of the lens which diminishes the vitality and resistance of the delicate lens fibres; formation of deposits between the lens fibres of acids and salts which have an irritating effect on the lens tissues and exert an increasing pressure on its delicate fibres, gradually destroying them; and disintegration of lens fibres, clouding the whole lens in the absence of appropriate measures.

Poisons in the blood stream due to dietetic errors and a faulty style of living can greatly contribute to the formations of cataract. The toxic matter in the blood stream spreads throughout the body to find shelter in any available weak spot. It strikes the lens if it has become weak through strain, excessive use of the eye and local irritation. The condition becomes worse with the passage of time and then a cataract starts developing. Other causes of cataract are stress and strain, excessive intake of alcoholic drinks, sugar, salt, smoking, certain physical ailments such as gastrointestinal or gall-bladder disturbances, diabetes, vitamin deficiencies, especially of

Vitamin C, fatty acid intolerances, radiation and side effects of drugs prescribed for other diseases.

Some specialists believe that the most important cause is poor nutrition. This may be true even in case of the type of cataract commonly called senile or ageing cataract. The cause may be a lifetime of malnutrition. Dr. Morgan Raiford, noted opthalmologist, who has studied cataracts for many years, considers faulty nutrition to be a basic factor in cataract.

Treatment

Cataract is one of the most stubborn conditions to deal with. If it has become deep-seated, nothing short of a surgical operation will help. However, in the early stages, there are good chances of getting over the ailment by natural means. Even advanced cases can be prevented from becoming worse.

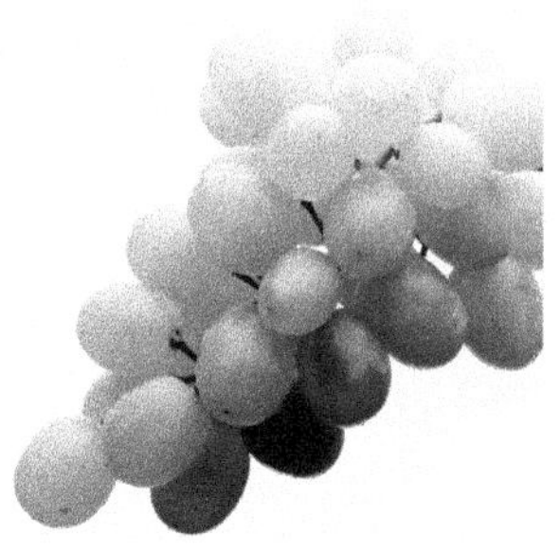

A thorough course of cleansing the system of the toxic matter is essential. To start with, it will be beneficial to undergo a fast for three to four days on orange juice and water. A warm water enema should be taken daily during this period. After this initial fast, a very restricted diet should be followed for two weeks. In this regimen, breakfast may consist of oranges or grapes or any other juicy fruit in season. Salads of raw vegetables in season, with olive oil and lemon juice dressing, and soaked raisins, figs or dates may be taken during lunch. Evening meals may consist of steamed vegetables such as spinach, fenugreek, drumsticks, cabbage, cauliflower, carrot, turnips (steamed in their own juices) and a few nuts or some fruits, such as apples, pears and grapes. Avoid potatoes and no bread or any other article of food should be added to this list.

After two weeks on this diet, the cataract patient may embark upon a fuller well-balanced diet — seeds, nuts, and whole grain cereals, vegetables and fruits. He may take fresh fruits, milk and a few nuts for breakfast; steamed vegetables, whole wheat chapattis and a glass of buttermilk for lunch; and a bowl of raw vegetable salad and sprouts for dinner.

The short fast followed by a restricted diet should be repeated after three months of the commencement of the treatment and again three months later, if necessary. The bowels should be cleansed daily with a warm water enema during the fast, and afterwards as necessary.

The patient should avoid white bread, sugar, cream, refined cereals, rice, boiled potatoes, puddings and pies, strong tea-coffee, alcoholic beverages, condiments, pickles, sauces, and other so-called aids to digestion.

There is increasing evidence to show that in several cases, cataracts have actually been reversed by proper nutritional treatment. However, the time needed for such treatment may extend from six months to three years.

Aniseed (saunf) is considered an excellent remedy for cataract. The patient should take about six grams aniseed and corriander powder, mixed with brown sugar is also beneficial. The mixture should be taken in doses 6 to 12 grams in morning and evening. Another valuable remedy for cataract is to grind seven kernels of almonds and half a gram of pepper together in water and drink it after sifting and sweetening the mixture with sugar candy. It helps the eyes to regain their vigour.

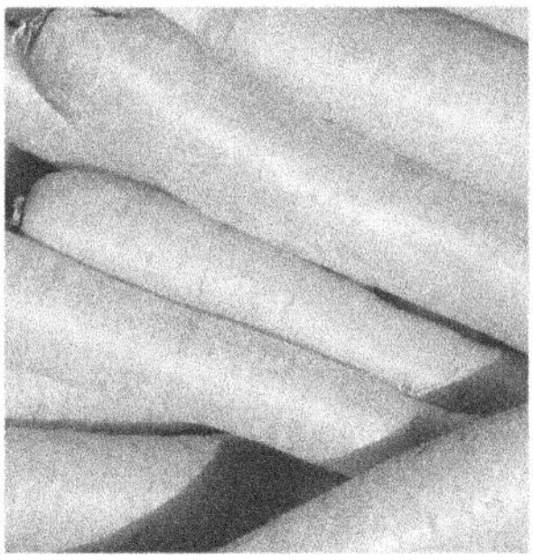

The use of carrots has been found valuable in cataract. The patient should eat plenty of raw carrots daily. Alternatively, he should take two glasses of carrot juice daily, one glass each morning and evening. Unprocessed honey has been found useful in treating cataract. A few drops of this honey should be put in the eyes. This is an ancient Egyptian remedy which has benefited many patients. The use of castor (arandi) oil has also been found beneficial. Two drops of this oil should be instilled in the eyes before retiring to bed.

The use of spinach is an effective home remedy to check cataract, according to a study in the British Medical Journal. A probable reason is spinach's rich stores of antioxidants, including beta carotene. Indeed, the investigators found that those who ate the most beta carotene in fruits and vegetables were only 40 per cent as likely to develop cataracts.

Simultaneous with the dietary treatment, the patient should adopt various methods of relaxing and strengthening the eyes. These methods have been explained earlier in Chapter 18 on low vision.

Epsom salt bath should also be taken twice a week. The procedure for this has been explained in the Appendix.

While fresh air and gentle outdoor exercise, such as walking, are other essentials, exposure to heat and bright light should be avoided.

CHAPTER 21

Glaucoma

Glaucoma is a serious eye condition characterised by an increase of pressure within the eye ball, called intraocular pressure. It is similar to high blood pressure in the body. The condition is also known as hypertension of the eye. A certain amount of intraocular pressure is considered necessary, but too much can cause damage to the eye and may result in vision loss.

The increase in the pressure results from buildup of fluid in the eye ball. This fluid nourishes the eyes and keeps them healthy. After the fluid circulates, it empties through a drain in the eye. In people with galucoma, the drain in the eye is blocked and the fluid cannot run out of the eyeball. Instead, it builds up and causes increased pressure in the eye.

Older persons are at greater risk of getting glaucoma than adults. However, in many cases the symptoms of the disease remain unnoticed until it is too late to prevent permanent handicap. The family history is the best guide to find out those at risk. All elderly persons whose parents, grandparents or other close relatives suffered from glaucoma are more at risk than others. All these people should undergo complete eye examination every year, to rule out the possibility of glaucoma, irrespective of the fact whether they have symptoms or not. Early detection of the disease can prevent damage to the eye's nerve cells and vision loss.

Symptoms

The first symptom of glaucoma is the appearance of halos or coloured rings round distant objects, when seen at night. In this condition, the iris is usually pushed forward, and the patient often complains of constant pain in the brow region, near the temples and the cheeks. Headaches are common. There is gradual impairment of vision as glaucoma develops, and this may ultimately result in blindness, if care is not taken to deal with the disease in the early stages.

Causes

Medical science regards severe eye strain or prolonged working under bad lighting conditions as the chief causes of glaucoma. But, in reality, the root cause of glaucoma is a highly toxic condition of the system due to dietetic errors, a faulty life style and the prolonged use of suppressive drugs for the treatment of other diseases. Eye strain is only a contributory factor.

Glaucoma is also caused by prolonged stress and is usually a reaction of adrenal exhaustion. The inability of the adrenal glands to produce aldosterone results in excessive loss of salt from the body and a consequent accumulation of fluid in the tissues. In the region of the eyes, the excess fluid causes the eyeball to harden, losing its softness and resilience. Glaucoma has also been associated with giddiness, sinus conditions, allergies, diabetes, hypoglycemia, arteriosclerosis and an imbalance of the autonomic nervous system.

Treatment

The modern medical treatment for glaucoma is through surgery which relieves the internal pressure in the eye due to excess fluid. This, however, does not remove the cause of the presence of the excess fluid. Consequently, even after the operation, there is no guarantee whatsoever that the trouble will not recur, or that it will not affect the other eye. The natural treatment for glaucoma is the same as that for any other condition associated with high toxicity and is directed towards preserving whatever sight remains. If treated in the early stages, the results are encouraging. Though cases of advanced glaucoma may be uncurable, certain nutritional and other biological approaches can prove effective in controlling the condition and preserving the remaining sight.

Certain foodstuffs should be scrupulously avoided by patients suffering from glaucoma. Coffee in particular should be completely avoided because of its high caffeine content. Caffeine causes stimulation of vasoconstrictors, elevating blood pressure and increasing blood to the eye. Beer and tobacco, which can cause constriction of blood vessels, should also be avoided. Tea should be taken only in moderation. The patient should not take excessive fluids, whether it is juice, milk or water at any time. He may drink small amounts several times with at least one-hour intervals.

The diet of the patient suffering from glaucoma should consist of seeds, nuts and grains, vegetables and fruit, with emphasis on raw Vitamin C-rich foods, fresh fruits and vegetables. Breakfast may consist of oranges or grapes or any other juicy fruits in season and a handful of raw nuts or seeds. Raw vegetables salad with olive oil and lemon juice dressing, two or three whole wheat chapattis and a glass of buttermilk may be taken for lunch. The dinner may comprise steamed vegetables, butter and cottage cheese.

Certain nutrients have been found helpful in the treatment of glaucoma. It has been found that the glaucoma patients are usually deficient in Vitamin A, B, C, protein, calcium and other minerals. Nutrients such as calcium and B-complex help relieve the intraocular condition. Many practioners believe that intraocular pressure in glaucoma can be lowered by the Vitamin C therapy. Dr. Michele Virno and his colleagues reported at a meeting of the Roman Ophthalmological Society in Rome, Italy, that the average person weighing 150 pounds who is given 7000 mg of ascorbic acid five times daily, acquired acceptable intraocular pressure within 45 days. Symptoms such as mild stomach discomfort and diarrhoea from large doses of Vitamin C were temporary and soon disappeared. It has also been suggested that some calcium should always be taken with each dose of ascorbic acid to minimise side effects of the large dose.

The patient should undertake various methods of relaxing and strengthening the eyes as explained in Chapter 18 on defective vision. He should avoid emotional stress and cultivate a tranquil, restful lifestyle. He should also avoid prolonged straining of the eye such as occurs during excessive T.V. or movie watching and excessive reading. The use of sunglasses should be avoided.

SECTION IV

CARDIOVASCULAR SYSTEM DISORDER

CHAPTER 22

Arteriosclerosis

Cardiovascular disease is the most common cause of death in old age. It is also the most important cause of ill health and disability in elderly people. There are certain effects of age on the cardiovascular system. Age-related changes in the cardiovascular systems include myocardial hypertrophy, with increased stiffness of the ventricles and thickening of the endocardium and valves. Myocardial contraction is prolonged, mainly due to slow relaxation. The resting stroke volume and cardiac output are reduced. However, the contractile ability of the myocardium is unchanged. The larger vessels become thickened and stiff.

Arteriosclerosis is one of the most common diseases of cardiovascular system. It refers to a thickening of the walls of the arteries due to the presence of calcium or lime. Arteriosclerosis is usually preceded by atherosclerosis, which is a universally prevalent disease in older people. It is a kind of degeneration or softening of the inner lining of the blood vessel walls. The most risky places for such degeneration are the coronary vessels of the heart and the arteries leading to the brain.

Arteriosclerosis results in the loss of elasticity of the blood vessels, with a narrowing of the smaller arteries, which interferes with the free circulation of the blood. These changes may gradually extend to capillaries and veins. Arteriosclerosis is the most important cause of cardiovascular disease in adults and majority of deaths from diseases related to arteriosclerosis occur in old people.

Symptoms

The symptoms of arteriosclerosis vary with arteries involved. Signs of inadequate blood supply generally appear first in the legs. There may be numbness and coldness in the feet and cramps and pains in the legs even after light exercise. If the coronary arteries are involved, the patient may have sharp pains, characteristic of angina pectoris. When arteries leading to the brain are involved, the vessel may burst, causing haemorrhage in the brain tissues. A cerebral vascular stroke, with partial or complete paralysis of side of the body may result, if there is blockage with a blood clot. It may also lead to loss of memory and a confused state of mind in elderly people. If arteries leading to the kidneys are involved, the patient may suffer from high blood pressure and kidney disorders.

Causes

The most important cause of arteriosclerosis is excessive intake of white sugar, refined foods and high fat diet, rich in cholesterol. Sedentary life and excesses of all kinds are the major contributing causes. Hardening of the arteries may also be caused by other diseases such as high blood pressure, obesity, diabetes, rheumatism, Bright's disease, malaria and syphilis. Emotional stress plays an important part, and heart attacks are more common during the periods of mental and emotional disturbances, particularly in those engaged in sedentary occupations. Heredity also plays its role and this disease runs in families.

Treatment

If the causes of arteriosclerosis are known, remedial action should be taken promptly to remove them. To begin with, the patient should resort to short juice fast for five to seven days. The juices of fresh raw vegetables and fruits may be taken diluted with water on 50:50 basis. Grapefruit, pineapple, lemon and juice of green vegetables are specially beneficial. A warm water enema should be used daily to cleanse the bowels during the period of juice fasting.

After that, the patient should take optimum diet consisting of seeds, nuts and grains, vegetables and fruits, with emphasis on raw foods and sprouted seeds. Vegetable oils like sunflower oil, flax seed oil and olive oil should be used regularly. Further short fasts on juices may be undertaken at intervals of three months or so, depending on the progress being made.

The patient should take several small meals instead of a few large ones. He should avoid all hydrogenated fats and an excess of saturated fats, such as butter, cream, ghee and animal fat. He should also avoid meat, salt and all refined and processed foods, condiments, sauces, pickles, strong tea, coffee, white sugar, white flour and all products made from them. Foods cooked in aluminum and copper utensils should not be taken as toxic metals entering the body are known to be deposited on the walls of the aorta and the arteries. Smoking, if habitual, should be given up because it constricts the arteries and aggravates the condition.

Recent investigations have shown that garlic and onions have a preventive effect on the development of arteriosclerosis. They should be included in the daily diet either raw or cooked.

One of the most effective home remedies for arteriosclerosis is the lemon peel. It strengthens the entire arterial system. Shredded lemon peel may be added to soups and stews, or sprinkled over salads. To make a medicine, the peel of one or two lemons may be cut up finely, covered with warm water and allowed to stand for about 12 hours. A teaspoonful may be taken every three hours, or immediately before or after a meal.

Parsley (Prajmoda) is another effective home remedy for this disease. It contains elements which help to maintain the blood vessels, particularly the capillaries and arterial system in a healthy condition. It may be taken as a beverage by simmering it gently in the water for a few minutes and partaking several times daily.

The beet juice has also proved valuable in arteriosclerosis. It is an excellent solvent for inorganic calcium deposits. Juices of carrot and spinach are also beneficial. These juices can be taken individually or in combination. Formula proportions found helpful when used in combination are 300 ml carrot and 200 ml spinach to prepare 500 ml of juice.

Honey is also considered beneficial in the treatment of arteriosclerosis. It is easily digested and assimilated. The patient should take a glass of water with one teaspoon each of honey and lemon juice in it, before going to bed. He can also take it if he wakes up at night.

The herb isabgol, botanically known as Plantagovata, has been found valuable in arteriosclerosis. The oil of the seeds of this plant should be used. It contains 50 per cent of linoleic acid, an unsaturated fat, and is, therefore, helpful in the prevention and treatment of this disease.

The patient should undertake plenty of outdoor exercise and eliminate all mental stress and worries. Prolonged neutral immersion baths at bed time on alternate days is beneficial. The procedure for taking this bath has been explained in Appendix.

CHAPTER 23

Coronary Heart Disease

The heart, the most vital organ in the body, is muscle about the size of a clenched fist. It is enclosed in a protective covering called the pericardium inside the chest. It starts working even before birth inside the womb. Weighing less than 350 grams, it pumps about 4,300 gallons of blood a day through the body and supplies oxygen and nourishment to all the organs. It beats 1,00,000 times a day, continuously pumping the blood through more than 60,000 miles of tiny blood vessels. The heart, in turn, needs blood for its nourishment which is supplied by coronary arteries.

A number of changes commonly occur in the heart in old age. The most important of these changes is rigidity of the myocardial wall due to an increase in collagen calcification of the ring of membranous valve between the left atrium and the left ventricle of the heart, known as mitral valves, and pulmonary valves. Other changes include some degree of muscle atrophy and the depositing of increasing amounts of age pigment lipofuscin. In the arteries thickening and fibrosis with resulting increased stiffness may cause a rise in systolic pressure with age and a fall in the diastolic pressure.

The term coronary heart disease covers a group of clinical syndromes arising particularly from failure of the coronary arteries to supply sufficient blood to the heart. They include angina pectoris, coronary thrombosis or heart attack and sudden death without infraction. There has been a marked increase in the incidence of heart disease in recent years. Heart attacks have become the biggest killer in Western countries. They rank third in India, after tuberculosis and infections.

In the event of narrowing or hardening of the arteries because of their getting plugged with fatty substances, the flow of blood is restricted. The heart then does not get sufficient oxygen. This condition is known as ischemia of the heart or angina pectoris. In this condition, exercise or excitement provokes severe chest pain and so limits the patient's physical activity. It serves as a warning to slow down and prompt preventive measures will prevent a heart attack. Angina is reported in about 10 per cent of people over 65 years old.

If the narrowed arteries get blocked due to a clot or thrombus inside them, causing death of that portion of the heart which depends on the choked arteries, it is called a heart attack or coronary thrombosis. It may lead to death or heal, leaving a scar. Patients with healed lesions may be severely disabled or may be able to resume normal life with restrictions in their physical activities.

Valvular disease of the heart is quite common in old age. Rheumatic heart disease accounts for a substantial proportion in old age while, congenital defects such as artial septal defects and aortic valve abnormalities may be encountered occasionally. Post mortem studies have shown that lesions are multiple and that few murmurs in the old are truly "insignificant".

Symptoms

A common symptom of heart disease is shortness of breath, which is caused by the blood being deprived of the proper amount of oxygen. Another common symptom is chest pain or pain down either arm. Other symptoms are palpitation, fainting, emotional instability, cold hands and feet, frequent perspiration and fatigue.

All these symptoms may also be caused by many other disorders. Appropriate tests and studies are, therefore, essential to establish the true nature of these symptoms.

Coronary thrombosis normally produces a severe chest pain which may last for at least half an hour. The pain may radiate down the left arm or up into the jaw. These symptoms are often absent in older patients. They may complain of breathlessness, palpitations, dizziness and general weakness. Often, they may quite suddenly become confused and depressed. Other old people with mental impairment may be unable to give a clear account of their symptoms. If there is a sudden deterioration in the health of an elderly patient, it is always advisable to consider the possibility of a coronary thrombosis.

Causes

The basic causes of heart disease are wrong feeding habits, faulty life style and various stresses. The famous Firamingham Heart Study of the National Heart and Lung Institute in Massachusetts identified seven major risk factors in coronary heart disease. These are: (i) elevated blood levels of cholesterol, triglycerides and other fatty substances, (ii) elevated blood pressure, (iii) elevated blood uric acid levels (mainly caused by high protein diet), (iv) certain metabolic disorders, notably diabetes, (v) obesity, (vi) smoking, and (vii) lack of physical exercise.

Each or combination of these risk factors can contribute to heart disease. Most of them are of dietary origin. These risk factors can be controlled by changing one's lifestyle and readjusting the diet. Constant worry and tension stimulate the adrenal glands to produce more adrenaline and cartisons. This also contributes to constricted arteries, high blood pressure and increased work for the heart. In the elderly, social and environmental factors also contribute greatly towards heart disease.

Treatment

The fundamental conditioning factor in all heart diseases is the diet. A corrective diet designed to alter body chemistry and improve the quality of general nutritional intake can, in many cases, reverse the degenerative changes which have occurred in the heart and blood vessels.

The diet should be lacto-vegetarian, low in sodium and calories. It should consist of high quality, natural organic foods, with emphasis on whole grains, seeds, fresh fruits and vegetables. Foods which should be eliminated are all white flour products, sweets, chocolates, canned foods in syrup, soft drinks, squashes, all hard fats of animal origin such as butter, cream and fatty meats. Salt and sugar should be reduced substantially. The patient should also avoid tea, coffee, alcohol and tobacco.

The essential fatty acids which reduce serum cholesterol levels and minimise the risk of arteriosclerosis can be obtained from sunflower seed oil and corn oil.

The use of olive oil is considered valuable in heart disease. It is dominant in mono-unsaturated fat. It lowers bad LDL cholesterol, but not good HDL cholesterol. It has antioxident activity which wards off artery damage from LDL cholesterol. In Italy, physicians use olive oil as a therapy after heart attack. Other important cholesterol lowering foods are alfalfa and yoghurt. Lecithin helps prevent fatty deposits in arteries. Best food sources are unrefined, raw, crude vegetable oils, seeds and grains.

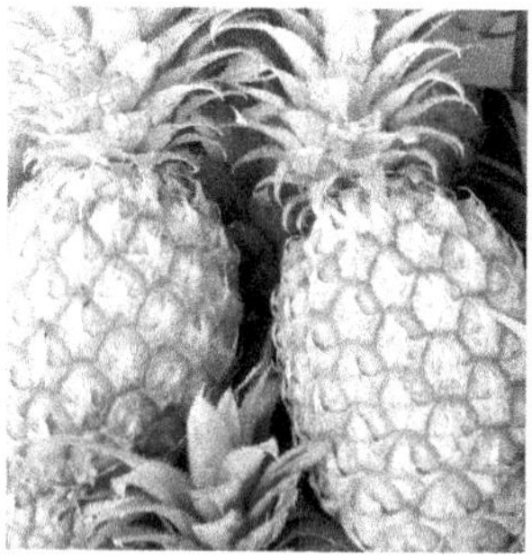

Fruits and vegetables in general are highly beneficial in the treatment of heart disease. Seasonal fruits are quite effective heart tonics. Apple contains heart stimulating properties and the patients suffering from the weakness of heart should make liberal use of the fruit. Fresh grapes, pineapple, orange, custard apple, pomegranate and coconut water also tone up the heart.

Grapes are effective in heart pain and palpitation of the heart and the disease can be rapidly controlled if the patient adopts an exclusive grapes diet for a few days. Grape juice, especially will be valuable when one is actually suffering from a heart attack. Indian gooseberry is considered an effective home remedy for heart disease. It tones up the functions of all the organs of the body, builds up health by destroying the heterogenous elements and renewing lost energy.

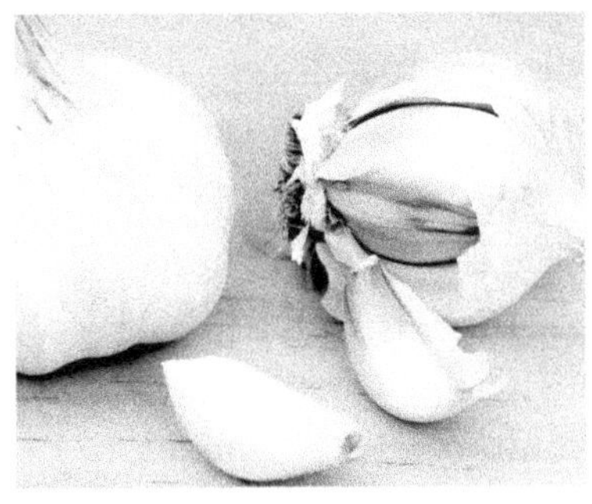

Another excellent home remedy for heart disease is garlic. Its regular use can even reverse the damage to arteries and help heal them. This conclusion has been reached by an Indian doctor, Arun Bordia of Tagore Medical College. He tested garlic on a group of 432 heart disease patients, recovering from heart attacks. Half the group ate two or three fresh raw or cooked garlic cloves every day for three years. They squeezed the garlic into juice, put it in milk as a "morning tonic" or ate it boiled or minced. The other half ate no garlic. After the first year, there was no difference in the rate of heart attacks between the groups.

In the second year, however, deaths among the garlic eaters dropped by 50 per cent and in the third year, they sank to 66 per cent! Non-fatal heart attacks also declined by 30 per cent in the second year and 60 per cent in the third year. Further, blood pressure and blood cholesterol in the garlic eaters fell about 10 per cent. Garlic eaters also had fewer attacks of angina — chest pain. There were no significant cardiovascular changes in the non-garlic eaters.

Dr. Bordia suggested that over time, steady infusions of garlic both wash away some of the arterial plaque and prevent future damage. Garlic's usefulness arises from the fact it contains 15 different antioxidents which may neutralize artery destroying agents.

The use of onions is also an effective home remedy for heart disease. They are useful in normalising the percentage of blood cholesterol by oxidising excess cholesterol. One teaspoon of raw onion juice first thing in the morning will be highly beneficial in such cases.

Honey has marvellous properties to prevent all sorts of heart disease. It tones up the heart and improves the circulation. It is also effective in cardiac pain and palpitation of the heart. One tablespoonful daily after food is sufficient to prevent all sorts of heart troubles.

Patients with heart disease should increase their intake of food rich in Vitamin E, as this vitamin promotes heart function by improving oxygeneration of the cells. It also improves the circulation and muscle strength. Many whole meal products and green vegetables, particularly outer leaves of cabbage are good sources of Vitamin E. The Vitamin B group is important for heart and circulatory disorders. The best sources of Vitamin B are whole grains.

Vitamin C is also essential as it protects against spontaneous breaches in capillary walls which can lead to heart attacks. It also guards against high blood cholesterol. The stress of anger, fear, disappointment and similar emotions can raise blood fat and cholesterol levels immediately but this reaction to stress can do little harm if the diet is adequate in Vitamin C and pantothenic acid. The richest sources of Vitamin C are citrus fruits.

The patient should also pay attention to other laws of nature for health building such as taking moderate exercise like walking, cycling, swimming and gardening, getting proper rest and sleep, adopting the right mental attitude and getting fresh air and drinking pure water.

Other useful methods in the treatment of heart disease are the use of an ice bag on the spinal area between the second and tenth thoracic vertebras for 30 minutes three times a week, a hot compress applied to the left side of the neck for 30 minutes every alternate day and massage of the abdomen and upper back muscles. Hot foot and hand baths are excellent for relieving the pain of angina pectoris.

Yoga can also help in alleviating heart diseases. Asanas such as shavasana, vajrasana and gomukhasana, yogic kriyas like jalaneti and pranayamas such as shitali, sitkari and bhramari are also helpful for heart ailments.

CHAPTER 24

Hypertension

Hypertension or high blood pressure, is regarded as the silent killer and is a disease of the modern age. The fast pace of life and the mental and physical pressures caused by the industrial and metropolitan environments give rise to psychological tensions. Worry and mental tension increase the adrenaline in the blood stream and this, in turn, causes the pressure of the blood to rise.

Hypertension is a common disease in old age and affects healthy people, too. Elevated blood pressure is a significant risk factor for both cardiovascular and cerebrovascular disease in old age. More than one-third of older people in the 65-74 age group have pressures greater than 160 mmHg systolic, and/or 95 diastolic. Blood pressure tends to rise with age, especially in an industralised society. Treating hypertension in old age therefore is of utmost importance in reducing morbidity and mortality.

The blood which circulates through the arteries within the body supplies every cell with nourishment and oxygen. The force exerted by the heart as it pumps the blood into the large arteries creates a pressure within them and this is called blood pressure. A certain level of blood pressure is thus essential to keep the blood circulating in the body. But when the pressure becomes too high, it results in hypertension which is caused by spasm or narrowing of the small blood vessels — capillaries throughout the body. This narrowing puts more stress on the heart to pump blood through the blood vessels. Hence, the pressure of the blood to get through rises in proportion to the pressure on the heart.

The blood pressure is measured in millimetres of mercury. The highest pressure reached during each heartbeat is called systolic pressure and the lowest between two beats is known as diastolic pressure. The first gives the pressure of the contraction of the heart as it pushes the blood on its journey through the body and indicates the activity of the heart The second represents the pressure present in the artery when the heart is relaxed and shows the condition of the blood vessels.

The blood pressure level considered normal is 120/70, but may go up 140/90 and still be normal. Within this range, the lower the reading, the better. Blood pressure between 140/90 and 160/95 is considered the borderline area. From 160/96 to 180/144, it is classed as moderate hypertension, while 180/115 and upward is considered severe. A raised diastolic pressure is considered more serious than the raised systolic pressure as it has a serious long-term effect.

It is not possible to describe a “normal” blood pressure in old age. The standards can be less stringent than in younger patients and a purely systolic hypertension is to be disregarded in practical terms although it is probably an indication of decreased vascular elasticity. A diastolic level of 110 mmHg or more can reasonably be taken as hypertensive if this is sustained under conditions which do not produce stress or anxiety. This rider is an important one because many old patients appear to have particularly unstable blood pressure. They may have high blood pressure readings when first examined or at casual readings, and be mistakenly diagnosed hepertensive, while regular daily charting of the blood pressure shows that the high early readings settle down to perfectly acceptable values after a few days.

Symptoms

Mild and moderate hypertension may not produce any symptoms for years. The first symptom may appear in the form of pain toward the back of the head and neck on waking in the morning, which soon disappears. Some of the other usual symptoms of hypertension are dizziness, aches and pains in the arms, shoulder region, leg and back, palpitations, pain in the heart region, frequent urination, nose-bleeding, nervous tension and fatigue, crossness, emotional upsets, tiredness and wakefulness.

An old person suffering from high blood pressure cannot do any serious work, feeling tired and out of sorts all the time. He may experience difficulty in breathing and suffer from dyspepsia. Hypertension, if not eliminated, may cause heart attacks or strokes and other disability conditions such as detachment of the retina.

Causes

The most important cause of hypertension is stress and a faulty lifestyle. People who are usually tense suffer from high blood pressure, especially when under stress. If the stress continues for a long period, the pressure may become permanently raised and may not come down even after the removal of the stress. An irregular lifestyle, smoking and an excessive intake of intoxicants, tea, coffee, cola drinks and refined foods destroy the natural pace of life. The expulsion of waste and poisonous matter from the body is prevented and the arteries and the veins become slack. Hardening of the arteries, obesity, diabetes and severe constipation also invite hypertension. Other causes of high blood pressure are excessive intake of pain-killers, common table salt, food allergies and eating a high-fat, low-fibre diet and processed foods deficient in essential nutrients.

Treatment

The natural way of dealing with hypertension is to eliminate the poisons from the system which cause it. The patient should always follow a routine of well-balanced diet, exercise and rest. Diet is of primary importance. The patient should start the process of healing by living on an exclusive fruit diet for at least five days and take fresh juicy fruits at five-hour intervals thrice in the day. Oranges, apples, pears, mangoes, pineapple, papaya and watermelon are the best diet in such cases. Milk may be added to the fruit diet after five days. The patient can be given cereals in his food after 10 days or so.

Vegetables are also good for a hypertension patient and vegetarians have strikingly lower blood pressure. Vegetables should preferably be taken raw. If they are cooked, it should be ensured that their natural juices are not burnt in the process of cooking. Vegetables like cucumber, carrot, tomato, onion, radish, cabbage and spinach are best taken in their raw form. They may be cut into small pieces with a little salt and the juice of a lemon added to them so as to make them more palatable. The intake of salt should be restricted; in any case it should not be taken more than four grams or half a teaspoon a day. Baking powder, containing sodium carbonate, should also be avoided.

Garlic is regarded as one of the most effective remedies to lower blood pressure. The pressure and tension are reduced because it has the power to ease the spasm of the small arteries. Garlic also slows the pulse and modifies the heart rhythm, besides relieving the symptoms of dizziness, numbness, shortness of breath and the formation of gas within the digestive tract. The average dosage should be two to three capsules a day to make a dent in the blood pressure. According to a researcher at George Washington University in America, both garlic and onion contain a great deal of adenosine which is a smooth muscle relaxant.

Celery (ajwain-ka-patta) is believed to have been used as folk remedy to lower blood pressure in Asia since 200 B.C. Dr. William Elholt, a pharmacologist at the University of Chicago's Pritzker

School of Medicine, has isolated a blood pressure reducing drug in this vegetable. The pressure lowering chemical is called 3-n-butylphthalide which gives celery its aroma. Dr. Elliot says celery may be unique because "the active blood pressure lowering compound is found in rather high concentrations in celery, and not in many other vegetables." He believes that the celery lowers pressure by reducing blood concentrations of stress hormones that cause blood vessels to constrict. He suggests celery may be most effective in blood pressure linked to mental stress. The patient can take two stalks of celery daily with beneficial results.

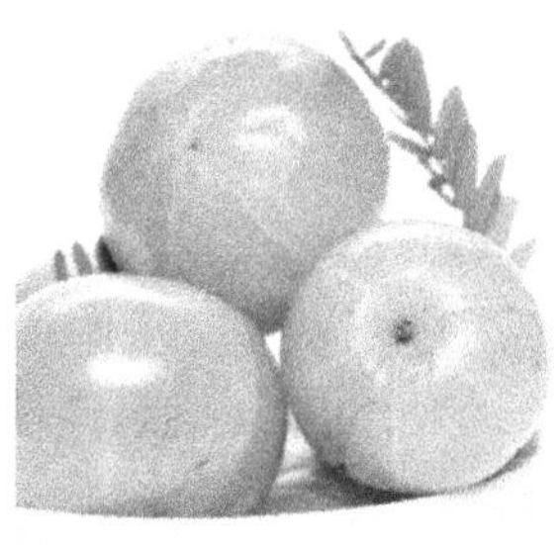

Indian gooseberry (amla) is another effective food remedy for high blood pressure. A tablespoon each of fresh amla juice and honey mixed together should be taken every morning in this condition. Lemon is also regarded as a valuable food to control high blood pressure. It is a rich source of Vitamin C which is found both in the juice and peel of the fruit. This vitamin is essential for preventing capillary fragility.

Watermelon is another valuable safeguard against high blood pressure. It was proved in recent experiments that a substance extracted from watermelon seeds has a definite action in dilating the blood pressure. The seeds dried and roasted should be taken in liberal quantities.

Potatoes, especially if boiled, are a valuable food for lowering blood pressure. When boiled with their skin, they absorb very little salt. Thus they can form a useful addition to salt-free diet recommended for patients with high blood pressure. Potatoes are rich in potassium but not in sodium salts. The magnesium present in the vegetable exercises beneficial effects in lowering blood pressure.

Recent studies have revealed an important link between dietary calcium and potassium, and hypertension. Researchers have found that people who take potassium-rich diets have a low incidence of hypertension even if they do not control their salt intake. They have also found that people with hypertension do not seem to get much calcium in the form of dairy products. The two essential nutrients seem to help the body throw off excess sodium and are involved in important functions which control the working of vascular system. Potassium is found in abundance in fruits and vegetables and calcium in dairy products.

The liberal use of Vitamin C in diet is also considered valuable in hypertension. According to Dr. Christopher Bulpitt, a hypertension expert at the Hammersmith Hospital in London, Vitamin C in fruits and vegetables is a powerful preventive medicine against blood pressure. He believes that high blood pressure and stroke fatalities are highest among people who eat the least Vitamin C. Researcher Paul Jacques in the U.S. Department of Agriculture's Human Nutrition Research Centre on Aging at Tufits University, says that a low intake of foods rich in Vitamin C predicts high blood pressure. In one study, he found that elderly people who ate Vitamin C in a single orange a day were twice as likely to have high blood pressure as those who ate four times that much. Systolic pressure was 11 points higher and diastolic pressure six points higher among the skimpy Vitamin C eaters. In another research, Dr. Jacques concluded that low blood levels of Vitamin C raised systolic pressure about 16 per cent and diastolic pressure 9 per cent.

The use of olive oil in diet may help lower blood pressure. A study by researchers at Stanford Medical School of 76 middle aged men with high blood pressure a few years ago concluded that the amount of monounsaturated fat in three tablespoons of olive oil a day could lower systolic pressure about nine points and diastolic pressure about six points. More remarkable, a University of Kentucky study found that a mere two-thirds of a tablespoon of olive oil daily reduced blood pressure by about five systolic points and four diastolic points in men.

The patient of hypertension should follow a plan of well balanced diet in which the constituents of food should be approximately in the following proportion: carbohydrate 20 per cent, protein 10 to 15 per cent, fat five per cent and fruits and vegetables 60 to 65 per cent. In this plan, one main meal should be based on raw foods, while the second main meal may consist of cooked foods. Meal should be taken slowly and in a relaxed atmosphere. Food should be well masticated as the process of digestion begins in the mouth. The dinner should not normally be taken late.

Exercise plays an important role in the treatment of hypertension. Walking is an excellent form of exercise. It helps to relieve tension, builds up the muscles and aids in the circulation of blood. As the blood pressure shows signs of abating, more exercise like bicycling, swimming and jogging should be taken. Yoga asanas such as vajrasana, padmasana, pavan-muktasana and shavasana and simple pranayama like anuloma-viloma and abdominal breathing are beneficial. All asanas should, however, be discontinued, except shavasana, if the blood pressure is above 200 mm.

Prolonged neutral immersion bath daily for an hour or so will work wonders. The procedure for taking this bath has been explained in Appendix.

CHAPTER 25

Varicose Veins

Veins are thin-walled vessels through which the impure blood is carried back to the heart. They usually have valves which regulate the flow of blood towards the heart. Varicose veins are veins have have become enlarged, dilated or thickened.

Varicose veins probably affect more than 10 per cent of the population, according to Dr. R.R. Footeos, Royal Waterloo Hospital, London, who has made a special study of this ailment quite common in old age.

Varicose veins can occur in any part of the body but generally appear on the legs. The veins of the legs are the largest in the body and they carry the blood from the lower extremities upwards towards the heart. The direction of circulation in these vessels is largely determined by gravity. Though there are no mechanical obstacles to blood flow, it is usually the incompetence of the valve which leads to an increase in intravenous pressure.

Varicose veins have an unsightly appearance and can be dangerous. A blood clot within a large, greatly dilated vein may break away and move towards the heart and lungs, causing serious complications.

Symptoms

The first sign of varicose veins is a swelling along the course of the veins. This may be followed by muscular cramps and a feeling of tiredness in the legs behind the knees. In some cases, the normal flow of blood towards the heart may be reversed when the patient is in an upright position. This results in veinous blood collecting in the lower part of the legs and the skin becomes purplish and pigmented, leading to what is known as varicose eczema or varicose ulcers. Both conditions cause severe pain.

Causes

A varicose condition of the veins results from sluggish circulation due to various factors such as constipation, dietetic errors, smoking and lack of exercise. Standing for long periods and wearing tight clothing can lead to sluggish circulation. Obesity can also cause varicose veins. Various emotional upsets, particularly suppressed anger, can make varicose veins worse. In such cases, large amounts of blood are still sent to the legs. When varicose veins exist, the return of this extra blood to the heart causes the already overloaded veins to swell further.

Treatment

For proper treatment of varicose veins, the patient should, in the beginning, be put on a juice fast for three to five days or on fruit diet for five to seven days. A warm-water enema should be administered daily during this period to cleanse the bowels and measures should be taken to avoid constipation.

After the juice fast or the fruits diet, the patient should adopt a restricted diet plan. In this regimen, oranges or orange and lemon juices may be taken for breakfast. The midday meal may consist of raw salad of any of the vegetables in season, with olive oil and lemon juice dressing. Steamed vegetables such as spinach, cabbage,

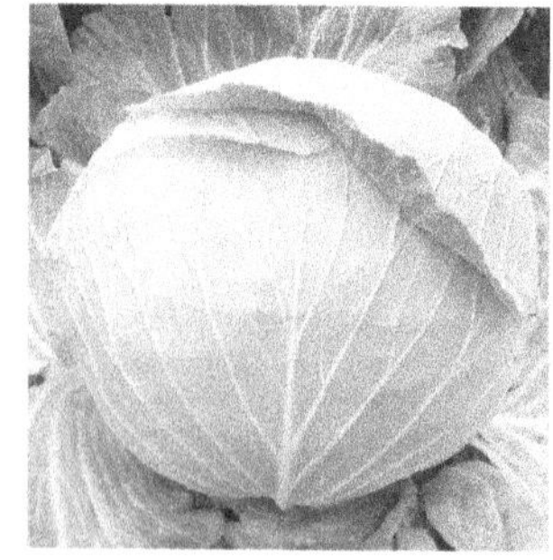

carrots, turnips, cauliflower and raisins, figs or dates may be taken in the evening. No bread or potatoes or other starchy foods should be included in this diet, or otherwise, the whole effect of the diet will be lost.

After the restricted diet, the patient may gradually embark upon a well-balanced diet with the emphasis on whole grains, seeds, nuts, vegetables and fruits. About 75 per cent of the diet should consist of raw vegetables and fruits. All condiments, alcoholic drinks, coffee, strong tea, white flour products, white sugar and white sugar products should be strictly avoided. A short fast or the fruit diet for two or three days may be undertaken every month, depending on the progress.

Raw vegetable juices, especially carrot juice in combination with spinach juice, have proved highly beneficial in the treatment of varicose veins. The formula proportions considered helpful in this combination are carrot 300 ml. and spinach 200 ml to prepare 500 ml. of juice.

Certain nutrients have been found effective in the treatment of varicose veins. The most important of these nutrients is Vitamin C. When Vitamin C is lacking, veins sag and become tortuous, which is the first stage of varicosity. In addition, there is often an anaemic condition present, which makes for a poor and weakened blood supply. Dr. Foote says, 'many of these patients are deficient in vitamins and healing may be accelerated by attention to this point, especially if large doses of Vitamin C are added to their diet.'

Also effective in treating this disease is Vitamin E. This vitamin is perhaps the most important nutrient for the health of blood vessels. According to Doctors Wilfiried and Evan Shute, in their article on Alpha Tocopherol (Vitamin E) in Cardiovascular Disease, a number of cases of what they describe as 'indolent ulcers', i.e., varicose ulcers, responded well to the use of Vitamin E. According to Dr. Shute, Vitamin E 'has an extraordinary ability to increase collateral circulation'. Thus, when a blood vessel is obstructed by a blood clot, Vitamin E helps to open up other blood vessels, to bypass the blood around the obstruction.

It does this by bringing into use the reserve network of veins that are always available for such an emergency. Vitamin E not only utilises these unused veins, but it has the property of enabling the tissues to make better use of oxygen, which is equivalent to an extra supply of blood to congested and devitalised areas. In addition, Vitamin E dissolves blood clots and strengthens muscular tissue.

Another vitamin which helps sufferers with varicose veins is Vitamin F (more often referred to as lecithin). The unbalanced modern diet is responsible for deposits of a hard, waxy substance called cholesterol being formed on the inner walls of veins and arteries, restricting the free flow of blood and causing blood vessels to harden and lose their natural resilience.

Lecithin emulsifies cholesterol and reduces it to tiny droplets that are readily assimilated and cannot form harmful deposits to clog the veins. Lecithin also helps the body to absorb Vitamin A, and it improves the body's utilisation of Vitamin E.

The alternate hot and cold hip bath will be very valuable and should be taken daily. The affected parts should be sprayed with cold water or cold packs should be applied to them. A mud pack may be applied at night and allowed to remain until morning. The hot epsom-salt bath is also very valuable and should be taken twice a week. The legs should be exposed to sunlight for some time during the day.

In case of varicose ulcers, packs, saturated with epsom salt, using one tablespoon of epsom salt to a glass of water, may be applied. The procedure is to wrap several folds of wet muslin cloth around the legs and covering them with at least two layers of dry fannel cloth, fastening all very comfortably. The alternate hot and cold leg bath is also beneficial in treating this condition. This bath is taken by immersing the legs alternatively in the hot and the cold water, one or two minutes in the hot water and one and a half or two minutes in the cold water. This treatment should be continued for 20 to 30 minutes once or twice a day until the ulcers are healed. After healing of the ulcers, the treatment may be used daily or two or three times a week as necessary. In painful varicose ulcers, ultraviolet radiation will be highly beneficial.

Precautionary Measures

Certain precautionary measures will help prevent varicose veins and ease symptoms, if the disease has already developed. These measures are as under:

(1) When on a long plane or train trip, get up and walk around every half an hour. If on a long trip by car, stop once in a while and get out to stretch your legs.

(2) When you are reading or watching television, elevate your feet and rest your legs on a chair or stool.

(3) Mobility helps general circulation. Walking is beneficial as the movements of leg muscles help push the blood upward. Swimming or walking in deep water against legs helps move the blood up the veins and protect against stagnation.

(4) Sleeping with feet raised slightly above the level of the heart helps the blood flow away from ankles. In case of serious trouble with varicose veins, the bed should be raised by placing blocks of six inches height under the posts at the foot. This is, however, not advisable for persons with heart trouble.

(5) If confined to bed, movement of feet and legs should be encouraged to help keep circulation moving youthfully.

(6) Round garters should never be worn. They cut off the venous circulation, thus raising pressure in the veins and increasing the risk of varicosities.

(7) Elastic girdles should not be worn continuously, especially

when seated for a long time, such as at a desk, or during a plane, train or auto trip. The girdles bunch up and hamper the return flow of blood.

Certain inverted yoga postures such as viparitakarani and sarvangasana are also beneficial in the treatment of varicose veins as they drain the blood from the legs and reduce pressure in the veins. They help to relax the muscles and allow the blood to flow freely in and out of the lower extremities. Padmasana, vajrasana and shalabhasana are also beneficial.

SECTION V

RESPIRATORY SYSTEM DISORDERS

CHAPTER 26

Pneumonia

Respiratory diseases are very common in old age. Age-related changes in respiratory system account for high incidence and prevalence of these diseases in the elderly. Pathologically, the lung in the elderly is lighter and shows loss of the elastic fibres which maintain the potency of small airways. This causes a progressive fall of vital capacity and of forced expiratory volume with age. There is also deterioration in lung compliance presumably due to such changes as calcification of the costal cartilages and arthritis of costo-vertebral joints leading to stiffening of the rib cage.

The elderly persons are particularly prone to respiratory infections which are a very important cause of both ill-health and death in old age. Nearly half of post-mortem examinations in elderly patients show bronchopneumonic changes of some degree. Investigations shows that the risk of death from pneumonia doubles every decade after the age of 20. Pneumonia, the acute inflammation of the lungs, is the most common infectious disease in the elderly. The disease is basically of two types, known as bronchopneumonia and lobar pneumonia.

Bronchopneumonia is an extension of infection from the bronchi to the substance of the lung, resulting in combined inflammation of the lung and the air passage. This type of pneumonia is quite frequent in old age. Response to treatment of bronchopneumonia in the elderly is not very encouraging, if the patient is in a debilitated condition. Although lobar pneumonia is considerably less common in old age than bronchopneumonia, it is of major occurrence in the elderly. Both the types of pneumonia often run into each other and are treated in the same way. The disease becomes more serious if both the lungs are affected. It is called double pneumonia in common parlance.

Symptoms

Most cases of pneumonia begin with a cold in the head or throat. The patient generally feels chill, shivering, difficulty in breathing and sharp pain in the chest, followed by a cough with pinkish sputum which may later become brownish. The patient usually suffers from fever and headache. In more serious cases, the sputum may be of rusty colour. Most patients feel very miserable and sweat profusely. The temperature may rise to 105°F and pulse may go upto 150 beats a minute. Primarily, bacterial pneumonia in the elderly may start with a distressing cough. Breathlessness and systemic symptoms may follow soon thereafter.

Causes

Pneumonia is caused by various types of germs such as streptococcus, staphylococcus and pneumococcus varieties. At times, certain viruses are also responsible for the disease. Other causes of this disease are fungal infection, irritation by worms, inhaling foreign matter, irritant dust or noxious gases and vapours such as ammonia, nitrogen dioxide or cadmium.

The real cause of pneumonia, however, is the toxic condition of the body, especially of the lungs and air passages, resulting from wrong feeding and faulty life style. Persons with healthy tissues and strong vital force are unlikely to catch pneumonia. It is only when the system is clogged with matter and the vitality is low that the germs of pneumonia invade a person.

Treatment

To begin with, the patient should be kept on a diet of raw juices for five to seven days, depending on the severity of the disease. In this regimen, he should take a glass of fruit or vegetable juice, diluted with warm water on 50:50 basis, every two hours. Fruits such as orange, sweet lime, apple, pineapple and grapes and vegetables like carrots and tomatoes may be used for juices.

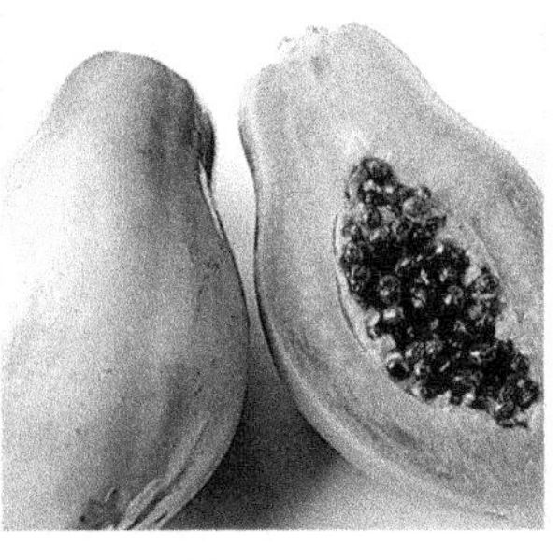

After a diet of raw juices, when the fever subsides, the patient should spend three or four further days on an exclusive fresh fruit diet, taking three meals a day of juicy fruits such as apple, grapes, pineapple, mango, orange, lemon and papaya. Thereafter, he may gradually adopt a well-balanced diet of natural foods consisting of seeds, nuts and grains, vegetables and fruits, with emphasis on fresh fruits and raw vegetables. The patient should be given warm water enema daily to cleanse the bowels during the period of raw juice therapy and all-fruit diet and thereafter, when necessary.

The patient should avoid strong tea, coffee, refined foods, fried foods, white sugar, white flour and all products made from them, condiments and pickles. He should also avoid all meats as well as alcoholic beverages and smoking. To reduce temperature naturally, during the course of the fever, full wet sheet pack may be applied as per procedure outlined in the Appendix.

Certain home remedies have been found beneficial in the treatment of pneumonia. During the early acute stage of this disease, herbal tea made from fenugreek (methi) seeds will help the body to produce perspiration, dispel toxicity and shorten the period of fever. It can be taken up to four cups daily. The quantity should be reduced as condition improves. To improve flavour, a few drops of lemon juice can be used. During this treatment, no other food or nourishment should be taken as fasting and fenugreek will help the body to correct these respiratory problems.

According to Dr. F. W. Crosman, an eminent physician, garlic is a marvelous remedy for pneumonia, if given in sufficient quantities. This physician used garlic for many years in pneumonia, and said that in no instance did it fail to bring down the temperature as well as the pulse and respiration, within 48 hours. Garlic juice can also be applied externally to the chest with beneficial results as it is an irritant and rubefacient.

Sesame seeds (til) are valuable in pneumonia. An infusion of the seeds, mixed with a tablespoon of linseed, a pinch of common salt and dessertspoon of honey, should be given in the treatment of this disease. This will help remove catarrhal matter and phlegm from the bronchial tubes.

The pain of pneumonia can be relieved by rubbing oil of turpentine over the rib cage and wrapping warmed cotton wool over it.

CHAPTER 27

Pulmonary Tuberculosis

Tuberculosis is one of the most serious infectious diseases. The World Health Organisation has described it as "humanity's greatest killer" and "the world's most neglected epidemic." Approximately 12 million people suffer from this disease all the world over at any given time and about three million of them die every year.

This disease is a major health problem in India and often rated the number one killer. This country accounts for about 40 per cent of the world's TB cases, and the health ministry has estimated that about six lakh people die of this disease every year.

Tuberculosis is of four types, namely of lungs, intestines, bones and glands. Pulmonary tuberculosis or tuberculosis of the lungs is by far the most common type of tuberculosis. It tends to consume the body.

Pulmonary tuberculosis is now primarily found in the elderly population. This age group still has a reservoir of mycobacteria which can become active during the period of growing old. It is also possible that the elderly person may have contracted the infection 50 or more years previously and diminished immunological defenses accompanying ageing and ill health may facilitate lung lesion, hitherto inactive, to break down and become reactivated.

The patient with pulmonary tuberculosis loses strength, colour and weight. Other symptoms are a rise in temperature hoarseness, difficulty in breathing, pain in the shoulders, indigestion, chest pain, and blood in the sputum.

The elderly patients may, however, not show the usual signs and symptoms attributable to tuberculosis. The disease may thus be overlooked in old age. More often, the patient merely feels vaguely unwell and this be wrongly attributed to ageing or depression. In many cases, the diagnosis is first recognised at post mortem. It is therefore always important to consider this diagnosis when the elderly persons complain of ill-health.

Causes

Tuberculosis is caused by a tiny germ called tubercle bacillus which is so small that it can be detected only by a microscope. The germ enters into the body through the nose, mouth and windpipe and settles down in the lungs. It multiplies by millions and produces small raised spots called tubercles. Those suffering from the disease for a considerable time eject living germs while coughing or spitting and when these germs enter the nose or mouth of healthy persons, they contract the disease. Mouth breathing and kissing as well as contaminated food and water are also responsible for spreading tuberculosis.

Lowered resistance or devitalisation of the system is, however, the real cause of this disease. This condition is brought about mainly by mineral starvation of the tissues of the body due to an inadequate dietary and the chief mineral concerned is calcium. In many ways, therefore, tuberculosis is the disease of calcium deficiency. There can be no breakdown of the tissue and no tubercular growth where there is adequate supply of organic calcium in the said tissue. Thus an adequate supply of organic calcium in the system together with organic mineral matter is a sure preventive of the development of tuberculosis.

Treatment

Tuberculosis is no longer considered incurable if it is tackled in the early stages. An all round scheme of dietetic and vitality building programme along natural lines is the only method to overcome the disease. As a first step, the patient should be put on an exclusive fresh fruit diet for three or four days. He should have three meals a day of fresh, juicy fruits, such as apples, grapes, pears, peaches, oranges and pineapple.

After the all-fruit diet, the patient should adopt a fruit-and-milk diet for four to six weeks. For this diet, the meals are exactly the same as the all-fruit diet, but with milk added to each fruit meal. The milk should be fresh and unboiled, but may be slightly warmed if desired. It should be sipped very slowly. Thereafter, the patient may adopt a well-balanced diet consisting of seeds, nuts and grains, vegetables and fruits.

The chief therapeutic agent needed for the treatment of tuberculosis is calcium. Milk, being the richest food source for the supply of organic calcium to the body, should be taken liberally. In the dietary outlined above, at least one litre of milk should be taken daily. Further periods on the exclusive fruit diet followed by a fruit-and-milk diet should be adopted at intervals of two or three months depending on the progress. During the first few days of the treatment, the bowels should be cleansed daily with the warm-water enema and afterwards as necessary.

The patient should avoid all devitalised foods such as white bread, white sugar, refined cereals, puddings and pies, tinned, canned and preserved foods. He should also shun strong tea, coffee, condiments, pickles and sauces.

The use of milk decoction with garlic has been found beneficial in the treatment of tuberculosis. Four cloves of garlic and one scraped coconut should be boiled in a litre of goat's milk till it is reduced to half. This milk, sweetened with honey, may be drunk early in the morning. This treatment should be continued for at least six weeks.

A tonic prepared from jackfruit (kathal) has been found valuable in tuberculosis. The edible portion of fully mature, but not fully ripe jackfruit, with the seeds intact, should be put in a glass container along with powdered jaggery. The two should be put in alternate layers. The top and bottom layers should be filled with jaggery. The container should be covered and placed in sunlight for 21 days. Thereafter, two or three teaspoons of this mixture should be taken three times daily. This treatment should be continued for at least three months.

The custard apple (sitaphal) is regarded as an effective food remedy for tuberculosis. It is said to contain the qualities of rejuvenating drugs. The Ayruvedic practitioners prepare a fermented liquor called sitaphalssava from the custard apple in its season for use as medicine in the treatment of tuberculosis. It is prepared by boiling custard apple pulp and seedless raisins in water on slow fire. It is filtered when about one-third of water is left. It is then mixed with powdered sugar candy along with the powder of cardamom, cinnamon and certain other condiments.

Indian gooseberry (amla) has proved another effective food remedy for tuberculosis. A tablespoon each of fresh amla juice and honey mixed together should be taken every morning in this condition. Its regular use will promote vigour and vitality in the body within a few days. Regular use of radish (muli) also helps.

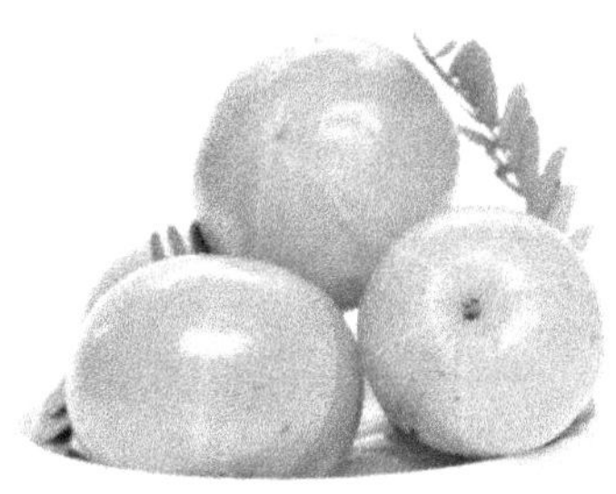

The patient should take complete rest relaxing both mind and body. Any type of stress will prevent healing. Fresh air is always important in curing the disease and the patient should spend most of the time in the open air and should sleep in a well-ventilated room. Sunshine is also essential as tuber bacilli are rapidly killed by exposure to sunrays. Other beneficial steps towards curing the disease are avoidance of strain, slow massage, deep breathing and light occupation to ensure mental diversion.

Certain yogic practices are also beneficial in the treatment of tuberculosis in its early stages. These include asanas like viparitakarni, sarvangasana, shavasana, jalneti kriya and anuloma-viloma pranayama.

CHAPTER 28

Bronchitis

Bronchitis refers to an inflammation of the mucous membrane lining the bronchi and bronchial tube within the chest. It is a breathing disorder affecting the respiratory function. In most cases, some infection also occurs in the nose and throat.

Bronchitis may be acute or chronic. In chronic cases, disease is of long duration. It is more serious than the acute type as permanent changes may have occurred in the lungs, thereby interfering with their normal movements. Chronic bronchitis is more frequent in males than in females. Mortality rate is also higher in males.

Acute bronchitis in the elderly usually occurs as an aggravation of chronic bronchitis and emphysema. Occasionally, it may also occur independently. Severe bronchitis in old age is infrequent, as severe cases die of this disease in late middle age and do not reach age group of elderly persons. However, the more modest degree of bronchitis is quite common in the elderly.

Symptoms

In most cases of bronchitis, the larynx, trachea and bronchial tubes are acutely inflamed. The tissues are swollen due to irritation. Large quantities of mucus are secreted and poured into the windpipe to protect the inflamed mucous membranes. The phlegm when expelled is found to be viscid and purulent. There is usually a high fever, some difficulty in breathing and a deep chest cough. Other symptoms are hoarseness and pain in the chest and loss of appetite. The breathing trouble continues till the inflammation subsides and mucus, is removed.

It sometimes becomes difficult to identify bronchitis in the elderly patients as many of them with clear sputum and no breathlessness do not seek medical advice. Simple tests of lung function are normal and so is the chest radiograph. Certain symptoms of bronchitis present in old age are mistakenly attributed to some other diseases in which these symptoms are also present.

Causes

The chief cause of bronchitis is wrong feeding habits. The habitual use of refined foods such as white sugar, refined cereals and white-flour products results in the accumulation of morbid matter in the system and collection of toxic waste in the bronchial tube. Another important cause of this disease is smoking. Excessive smoking irritates the bronchial tubes and lowers their resistance so that they become vulnerable to germs breathed in from the atmosphere. Other causes of bronchitis are living or working in stuffy atmospheres, use of drugs to suppress earlier diseases and hereditary factors, changes in weather and environment are common factors for the onset of the disease.

Treatment

In acute cases of bronchitis, the patient should fast on orange juice and water till the acute symptoms subside. The procedure is to take juice of an orange in a glass of warm water every two hours from 8 a.m. to 8 p.m. During this period, a warm water enema should be administered daily to cleanse the bowels. After the juice fast, the patient should adopt an all-fruit diet for further two or three days. In case of chronic bronchitis, the patient can begin with an all-fruit diet for five to seven days, taking three meals a day of fresh juicy fruits such as orange, apple, pineapple, grapes and papaya.

After the all-fruit diet, the patient should follow a well-balanced diet consisting of seeds, nuts and grains, vegetables and fruits. For drinks, unsweetened lemon water or cold or hot plain water may be taken. The patient should avoid meats, sugar, tea, coffee, condiments, pickles, refined and processed foods, soft drinks, candies, ice-cream and products made from sugar and white flour. The elderly patient should be persuaded to give up smoking as the habit still persists in old age and exercises adverse effects.

One of the most effective remedies for bronchitis is the use of turmeric (haldi) powder. A teaspoonful of this powder should be administered with a glass of milk two or three times daily. It acts best when taken on an empty stomach.

Another effective remedy for bronchitis is mixture of dried ginger powder, pepper and long pepper (pipli) taken in equal quantities, three times a day. It may be licked with honey. The powder of these three ingredients have antipyretic qualities and are effective in dealing with fever accompanied with bronchitis. They also tone up the metabolism of the patient.

Onion has been used as a food remedy for centuries in bronchitis. It is said to possess expectorant properties. It liquefies phlegm and prevents its further formation. One teaspoon of raw onion juice first thing in the morning will be highly beneficial in such cases.

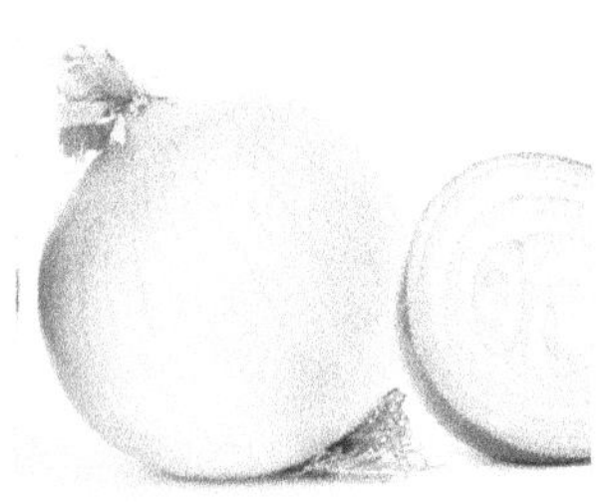

The liberal use of Vitamin C rich foods has been found valuable in the prevention and treatment of bronchitis. Vitamin C is considered cell protective antioxidant. Food rich in this vitamin can therefore help protect the lungs from damage and consequent debilitating bronchitis. In a major study of 9,000 patients, Dr. Joel Schwartz of the U.S. Environmental Protection Agency, discovered that people who ate foods containing 300 mg of Vitamin C a day were only 70 per cent as likely to have chronic bronchitis or asthma as those eating foods with one-third that much or about 100 mg. The difference of 200 mg of Vitamin C can be obtained from two glasses of orange juice.

Dr. Schwartz says that a Vitamin C rich diet is especially valuable for cigarette smokers who are at high risk for chronic obstructive bronchitis, if they smoke long enough. Investigations show that smokers use up Vitamin C rapidly to counteract the toxic oxidative agents in cigarette smoke. They therefore need approximately three and half times more Vitamin C than non-smokers. Foods rich in Vitamin C are citrus fruits, Indian goosebery (amla), green leafy vegetables and sprouted Bengal and green grams.

Simple hot poultice of linseed should be applied over the front and back of the chest. It will greatly relieve pain. These poultices act by diluting the vessels of the surface and thereby reducing the blood pressure. The heat of the poultice acts as a cardiac stimulant. The poultice should be applied neatly and carefully and should be often removed, so that it does not hamper respiration. Turpentine may be rubbed over the chest with fomentation for the same object.

A hot epsom-salts bath every night or every other night will be highly beneficial during the acute stages of the attack. The procedure for preparing this bath has been explained in the Appendix. In case of chronic bronchitis, this bath may be taken twice a week. Hot towels wrung out and applied over the upper chest are also helpful. After applying three hot towels in turn for two or three minutes each, one should always finish off with a cold towel. A cold pack should also be applied to the upper chest several times daily in acute conditions. The procedure for application of this pack has been explained in Appendix.

Fresh air and outdoor exercises are also essential to the treatment of bronchitis and the patient should take a good walk every day. He should also perform yogic kriyas such as Jalneti and vamandhouti and yogic asanas such as ekpaduttanasana, yogamudra, bhujangasana, shalabhasana, padmasana and shavasana. Simple pranayams like kapalbhati, anuloma-viloma, ujjayi and bhramari will also be very useful.

CHAPTER 29

Emphysema

Emphysema is a serious and debilitating lung disease. In this condition, alveoli, the tiny air sacs in the lungs and bronchioles, the narrow passages leading to the air sacs, become permanently distended with air. The lung tissues lose their elasticity, and the number of blood vessels is reduced. It is essentially a chronic disease, which generally occurs after the age of 40. It is less frequent in women.

Severe type of emphysema is rare in old age. This is because severe cases generally occur in middle age and most often prove fatal by the time patient reaches late middle age. However, more modest degree of emphysema is common in the elderly and the clinical picture of the disease is similar to that in middle age.

Symptoms

The main symptoms of emphysema is breathlessness followed by coughing. It gets worse with the lapse of time. Eventually the patient is breathless at rest, as the alveoli becomes so damaged that the exchange of gases between the blood and the air is much impaired. The patient feels difficulty in chewing and swallowing due to breathlessness. There may be discomfort after a meal because the lungs have expanded, pushing the diaphragm into the stomach. Other symptoms are loss of appetite and weight loss.

In severe cases, the chest itself may get enlarged and the movement of the ribs may diminish. The volume of air passed in and out of the lungs at each breath becomes very much less than normal.

Causes

Emphysema is frequently found in association with asthma and chronic bronchitis. Obstruction of the air passages and infection are thus the main factors which bring about this disease. This weakens the elastic tissues of the lungs. Other causes of emphysema are continuous exposure to dust and high levels of air pollution. Smoking is also an important contributory factor.

Treatment

To begin with, the patient should undertake a fast on fruits or vegetable juices for about five days. During this period, a warm-water enema should be used daily to cleanse the bowels. The juice fast may be followed by an exclusive diet of fresh juicy fruits such as apple, pineapple, pear, peach, orange and papaya for further five days or so.

The patient may thereafter gradually adopt a well-balanced diet of seeds, nuts and grains, vegetables and fruits. The diet should be supplemented with vegetables oil, honey and goat's milk, preferably in soured form like curd and buttermilk. The emphasis should be on fresh fruits and raw vegetables, as well as fruit and vegetable juices. The short juice fast followed by an all-fruit diet may be repeated at intervals of two months or so depending on the condition.

Among home remedies is the use of garlic. Two or three cloves of this vegetable should be chewed daily, preferably in the morning on an empty stomach. A little, garlic juice can also be added to vegetable juices.

The use of lemon or lime is another valuable home remedy for emphysema. A teaspoon of fresh juice of either of the two fruits should be taken several times a day before or between meals.

Amaranth (chaulai-ka-saag) has proved beneficial in the treatment of this disease. Fresh juice should be extracted from this green leafy vegetable. This juice should be mixed with honey and drunk liberally by the patient.

The aniseed (saunf) has also been found valuable in emphysema due to its expectorant properties. Five to ten drops of aniseed oil should be mixed with one teaspoon of brown sugar. This mixture can be taken with beneficial results in treating this disease. It is an old emphysema 'cure' in folk medicine.

Raw juices of fresh fruits and vegetables have been found beneficial in the treatment of emphysema and the patient should make liberal use of these juices. Vegetables which can be used for juices are green vegetables, carrot, water-cress and raw potato. Fruits which can be used for juices are lemon, orange and pineapple.

The use of salt in the diet should be restricted as the normal intake of salt is harmful for emphysema patient. According to Dr. Joel Schwartz of the U.S. Environmental Protection Agency, a high-salt diet can cause emphysema and other respiratory diseases. The reason is that too much sodium throws the sodium-potassium ratio out of balance, setting off an exaggerated response by bronchial passages as well as by nervous system controls that lead to inflammation and lung damage.

The patient should live in a place, with the least air pollution and smoke-free environment. The chronic bronchitis which is associated with emphysema must be kept under control as far as practicable through natural methods of treatment. Smoking, if habitual, should be given up. Breathing pure oxygen from a cylinder will allow enough of the gas to enter the blood. Weight loss can be overcome by taking frequent small meals comprising high energy foods.

The patient should undertake mild exercises which will help maintain muscle tone and prevent them from becoming rigid. Walking is especially beneficial and the patient should walk for at least five kms. morning and evening daily. He should also undertake deep breathing exercises in fresh air.

CHAPTER 30

Asthma

Asthma is an allergic condition resulting from the reaction of the system to one or more allergens. It is the most troublesome of the respiratory diseases. The asthma patient gets frequent attacks of breathlessness, in between which, he is completely normal.

This disease is quite common and it is estimated that approximately 2.5 per cent of population suffer from bronchial asthma. About 65 per cent of these patients develop the symptoms in early young age. The disease is more common in advanced, industrialised countries than in primitive, tribal communities. It is found more in men than in women.

Asthma is an ancient Greek word meaning "panting or short drawn breath." Patients suffering from this disease appear to be gasping for breath. Actually, they have more difficulty in breathing out than breathing in and it is caused by spasm of the smaller air passage in the lung. The effect is to blow the lungs up because the patient cannot drive the air properly out of the lungs before he has to take another breath.

Symptoms

The onset of asthma is either abrupt or gradual. Sudden onsets are often preceded by a spell of coughing. When the onset is gradual, the attack is usually brought on by respiratory infection.

A severe attack causes an increase in heartbeat and respiratory rates and the patient feels restless and fatigued. There may be coughing, tightness in the chest, profuse sweating and vomiting. There may also be abdominal pain, especially if coughing is severe. The wheezing sound identified with asthma is produced by the air being pushed through the narrowed bronchi. All asthmatics have more difficulty at night, especially during sleep.

In the elderly, the recurring periods of distressing and often nocturnal cough, may occur after an upper respiratory infection. It suggests late onset of asthma. Wheezing, if not the original complaint, will often have been noticed by the patient or his spouse. The lungs may appear normal when examined during the day, but serial measurements of peak expiratory flow rate several times a day and at night if woken by cough, will normally show the wide fluctuations characteristic of asthma.

Causes

Asthma is caused by a variety of factors. For many, it is an allergic condition resulting from the reaction of the system to the weather, food, drugs, perfumes and other irritants which vary with different individuals. Allergies to dust are the most common. Some persons are sensitive to the various forms of dust like cotton dust, wheat dust and paper dust, some pollens, animal hair, fungi and insects, especially cockroaches. Foods, which generally cause allergic reactions are wheat, eggs, milk, chocolates, beans, potato, pork and beef.

For others, asthma may result from the abnormal body chemistry involving the system's enzymes or a defect in muscular action within the lungs. Quite often, however, it is precipitated by a combination of allergic and non-allergic factors, including emotional tension, air pollution, infections and hereditary factors. It has been estimated that when both parents have asthma or hay fever, in 75 to 100 per cent cases, the offspring also has allergic reactions.

It is difficult to identify any avoidable external cause for asthma in the elderly, but all efforts, should be made to do so. Enquiries should be made about exposure to animals, chemicals or organic dusts. It is also important to ensure that the patient is not taking drugs that may cause or increase airflow obstruction.

Treatment

Modern medical system has not been able to find a cure for this crippling disease. Drugs and vaccines have only limited value in alleviating the symptoms. Most of these are habit forming and the dose has to be increased from time to time to give the same amount of relief. The frequent introduction of drugs in the system, while giving only temporary relief, tends to make asthma chronic and incurable. Allergy, which is the immediate cause of asthma, itself is an indication of lowered resistance and internal disharmony caused by faulty eating and bad habits. This is the root cause and the real cure lies in a return to nature.

The natural way to treat asthma consists of stimulating the functioning of slack excretory organs, adopting appropriate diet patterns to eliminate morbid matter and reconstruct the body, and practising yogasanas, yogic kriyas and pranayamas to permit proper assimilation of food and to strengthen the lungs, digestive system and circulatory organs.

The patient should be given an enema to clean the colon and prevent auto-intoxication. Mud-packs applied to the abdomen will relieve the fermentation caused by undigested food and will promote intestinal peristalsis. Wet packs should be applied to the chest to relieve the congestion of the lungs and strengthen them. The patient should be made to perspire through steam bath, hot foot bath, hot hip bath and sun bath. This will stimulate the skin and relieve congested lungs.

The patient should fast for a few days on lemon juice with honey and thereafter resort to a fruit juice diet to nourish the system and eliminate the toxins. Solid foods can be included gradually. The patient should, however, avoid the common dietic errors. Ideally, his diet should contain a limited quantity of carbohydrates, fats and proteins which are acid-forming foods, and a liberal quantity of alkaline foods consisting of fresh fruits, green vegetables and germinated gram. Foods which tend to produce phlegm such as rice, sugar, lentils and curds as also fried and other difficult-to-digest foods should be avoided.

Asthmatics should always eat less than their capacity. They should eat slowly, chewing their food properly. They should drink eight to 10 glasses of water a day, but should avoid taking water or any liquid with meals. Spices, chillies and pickles, too much tea and coffee should also be avoided.

Asthma, particularly when the attack is severe, tends to destroy the appetite. In such cases, do not force the patient to eat. He should be kept on fast till the attack is over. He should, however, take a cup of warm water every two hours. An enema taken at that time will be very beneficial.

Eating the right foods may alleviate or prevent asthmatic attack by helping control underlying inflammation of air passages, dilating air passages, thinning down mucus in the lungs and preventing food allergy reactions that trigger asthma attacks.

Eating onion regularly is one of the most effective remedies for asthma. A prominent researcher in the field, Dr. Walter Dorsch of Johannes-Guttenberg University in Mainz, Germany, has discovered strong anti-inflammatory activity in both onion juice and specific onion compounds. In one such test, an onion chemical diphenylthiosulphinate displayed higher anti-inflammatory activity than the popular anti-inflammatory drug prednisolone.

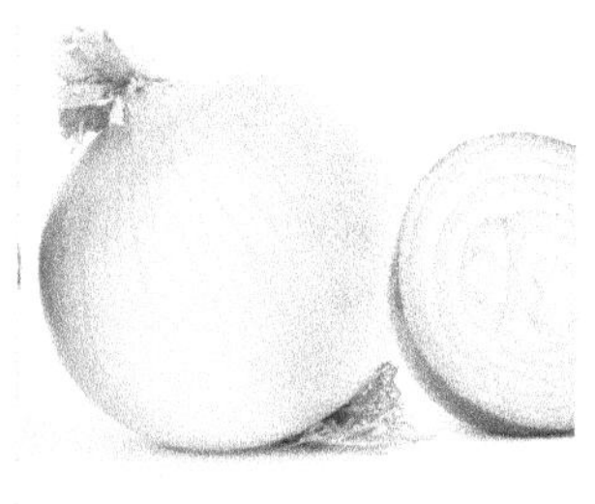

Dr. Dorsch has found that onions do have direct anti-asthmatic effects. He credits thiosulphinates in onions as the major active anti-inflammatory agents. However, onions are the richest of all foods in another powerful anti-inflammatory compound, quercetin, which also can relieve allergies.

Eating hot pungent foods can give immediate relief from asthma. According to Dr. Irwin Ziment, a pulmonary disease expert, hot chilli pepper, spicy mustard, garlic and onions can all make breathing easier for asthmatics by opening up air passage. He explains that such foods have mucus moving activity that thins out the viscous mucus which otherwise would plug up the small airways, making breathing difficult for asthmatics. Dr. Ziment believes that spicy foods stimulate nerve endings in the digestive tract which releases watery fluids in the mouth, throat and lungs. These secretions help thin down the mucus, so it does not clog airways and can be expelled, allowing normal breathing.

Honey is considered beneficial in the treatment of asthma. It is said that if a jug of honey is held under the nose of an asthma patient and he inhales the air that comes into contact with the honey, he starts breathing easier and deeper. The effect lasts for about an hour or so. This is because honey contains a mixture of 'higher' alcohols and ethereal oils and the vapours given off by them are soothing and beneficial to the asthma patients. Honey usually brings relief whether the air flowing over it is inhaled or whether it is eaten or taken either in milk or water. It thins out accumulated mucus and helps its elimination from the respiratory passages. It also tones up the pulmonary parenchyma and thereby prevents the production of mucus in future.

Another effective remedy for asthma is garlic. The patient should be given daily garlic cloves boiled in 30 gms milk as a cure for early stages of asthma. Steaming ginger tea with minced garlic cloves in it, can also help to keep the problem under control and should be taken both in the morning and evening. Turmeric is also

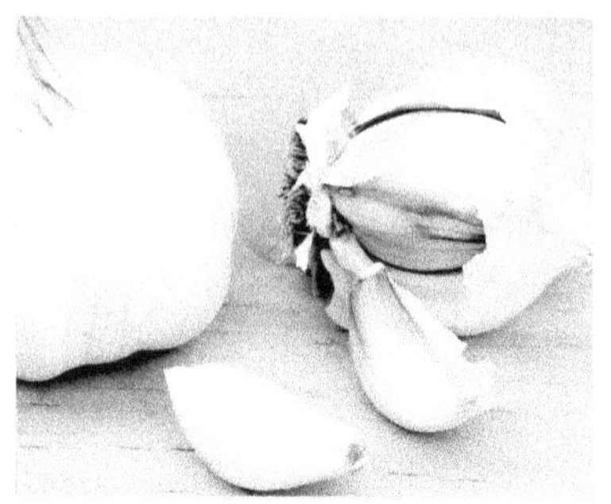

regarded as an effective remedy for bronchial asthma. The patient should be given a teaspoon of turmeric powder with a glass of milk two or three times daily. It acts best when taken on an empty stomach.

During the attack, mustard oil mixed with little camphor should be massaged over the back of the chest. This will loosen up phelgm and ease breathing. The patient should also inhale steam from the boiling water mixed with caraway seeds (ajwain). It will dilate the bronchial passage. The patient should also follow the other laws of Nature. Air, sun and water are great healing agents. Regular fasting once a week, an occasional enema, breathing exercises, fresh air, dry climate, light exercises and correct posture go a long way in treating the disease.

The patient should perform yogic kriyas such as jalneti, vamandhouti and yogic asanas such as ekapadauttanasana, yogamudra, sarvangasana, padmasana, bhujanagasana, dhanurasana, vakrasana, shalabhasana. paschimottanasana and shavasana, Pranayamas like kapalbhati, anuloma-viloma, ujjayi and bhramari will also be highly beneficial.

The patient should avoid dusty places, exposure to cold, foods to which he is sensitive, mental worries and tensions.

CHAPTER 31

Cough

The air passages of the lungs are lined with cells secreting mucus, which normally traps particles of dust. When the membranes are infected and inflamed, the secretion of mucus increases and the lining of air passages is irritated. Coughing is the action by which excess mucus is driven out. In the process, a dry hacking sound is produced. It is a very common condition affecting persons of all ages especially the older age group. Cough in the elderly may be either of recent origin or long standing.

Coughing is a vital body defense mechanism. It ejects everything from germs to foreign bodies from the lungs and windpipe. When a person is unable to cough which may happen, for instance, following surgery or a chest injury, pneumonia can become a serious threat.

Symptoms

First, a person who is going to cough draws a deep breath in. He then closes his glottis and contracts his muscles. This builds up pressure in the chest. Then, he suddenly opens his glottis so that there is an explosive discharge of air which sweeps through the air passages and carries with it the excess secretions or, in some cases, foreign matter which has irritated the larynx, trachea or bronchi.

Causes

Cough may be caused by inflammation of the larynx or the pharynx. It may also be caused by digestive disturbance. A cough can develop in the chest due to weather condition or seasonal changes. The real cause of this disorder, however, is clogging of the bronchial tube with waste matter. This has been brought about by wrong feeding habits. The reason for higher incidence of cough during winter than in other seasons is that an average person usually eats more of the catarrh-forming foods such as white bread, meat, sugar, porridge, puddings and pies in the colder months of the year. Overclothing with heavy undergarments during this period also prevents proper aeration of the skin.

Cough of recent onset in the elderly may result from acute infection, asthma, lung tumour, tuberculosis and breathing of foreign body. Long-standing cough may be caused by chronic bronchitis, bronchiectasis, tuberculosis, lung tumour and breathing of oesophageal contents. Cough of recent origin in the elderly is most commonly associated with respiratory infection, the overwhelming majority of which are viral. Recurring periods of distressing cough, especially in the night, may occur after an upper respiratory infection.

Treatment

In case of severe cough, the patient should take only orange juice and water till the severity is reduced. The procedure is to take the juice of an orange diluted in warm water every two hours from 8 a.m. to 8 p.m. The patient should drink hot water freely. This will make the secretion thinner and less viscid, thereby loosening the cough. The quantity of water should be considerable so as to cause a feeling of warmth and perspiration, giving much relief. The warm water enema should be used daily to cleanse the bowels. After the juice diet, the patient should adopt an all-fruit diet for two or three more days.

In case of mild cough, the patient can begin with an all-fruit diet for five to seven days, taking three meals a day of fresh juicy fruits such as apples, pears, grapes, grape-fruit, oranges, pineapple, peaches and melon. For drinks, unsweetened lemon water or cold or hot plain water may be taken. After the all fruit diet, the patient should follow a well-balanced diet, with emphasis on whole grain cereals, raw or lightly-cooked vegetables and fresh fruits.

The patient should avoid meats, sugar, tea, coffee, condiments, pickles, refined and processed foods. He or she should also avoid soft drinks, candies, ice-cream and all products made from sugar and white flour.

One of the most effective home remedies is the use of grapes. They tone up the lungs and act as an expectorant. Simple cold and cough are relieved through its use in a couple of days. A combination of honey with grape juice is specific for cough.

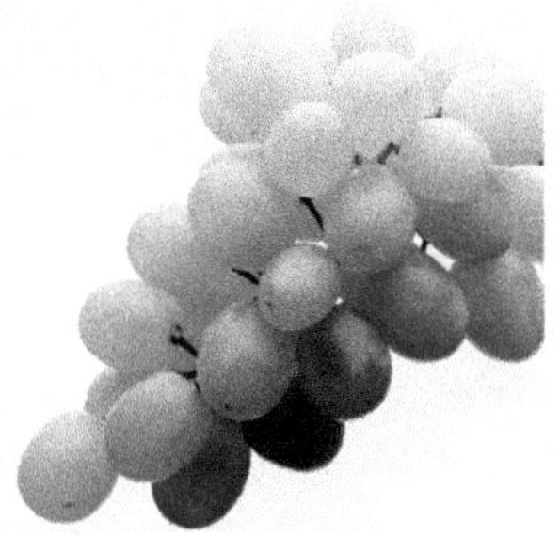

Almonds (badam) are useful in dry coughs. They should be soaked in water for about an hour or so and the brown skin removed. They should then be ground well to form a fine paste and 20 grams each of butter and sugar added to it. This paste should be given in the morning and evening.

Onion (Piyaz) is valuable in cough. This vegetable should be chopped fine and juice extracted from it. This juice mixed with honey and kept for four or five hours will make an excellent cough syrup. It is also useful in removing phlegm. A medium size onion should be crushed, the juice of one lemon should be added to it, and then one cup of boiling water should be poured on it. Some honey should be added for taste and it should be taken two or three times a day.

The root of turmeric (haldi) plant is useful in dry cough. The root should be roasted and powdered. This powder should be taken in three gram doses twice daily in the morning and evening.

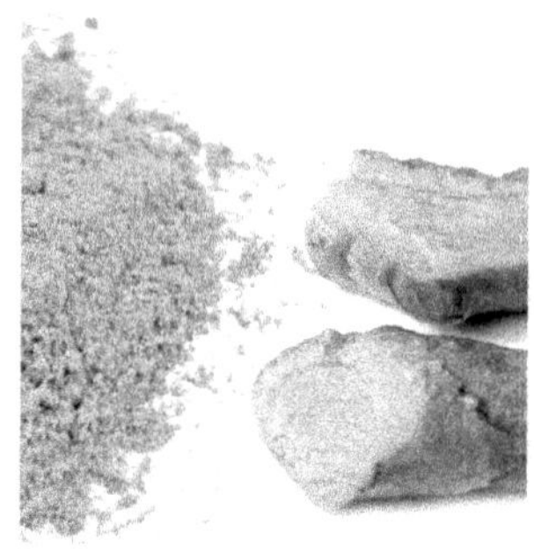

The herb belleric myroblan (bahera) is a household remedy for cough. A mixture of the pulp of the fruit, long pepper and honey should be administered for the treatment of this condition. The dried fruit covered with wheat flour and roasted, is another popular remedy for cough condition.

A sauce made from raisins (munaqqa) is valuable in cough. This sauce is prepared by grinding 100 grams of raisins with water. About 100 grams of sugar should be mixed with it and the mixture should be heated and preserved when the bulk has turned saucy. This sauce should be taken in 20 grams dose at bed time daily.

Aniseed (vilaiti saunf) is also useful in hard dry cough with difficult expectoration. It breaks up mucus. A tea made from this spice should be taken regularly for treating this condition.

Other measures

Other useful measures in the treatment of cough are hot fomentations to the chest and throat and application of frequent chest packs. If the cough is checked while the secretion is abundant, the patient should be made to sit in the tub with a small amount of hot water, and cold water should be poured over his head, spine and chest to induce cough. This should be followed by vigorous rubbing. The patient should be dried thoroughly and then wrapped in dry blankets in the bed.

SECTION VI

DISEASES OF THE GASTROINTESTINAL SYSTEM

CHAPTER 32

Hiatus Hernia

A number of age changes occur in the gastrointestinal tract. These include deterioration in esophageal motility, prolongation of gut transit time and a consequent possibility of developing constipation. Many pathological conditions may also commonly affect the elderly.

Hiatus hernia is the most common disease of the gastro-intestinal system in old age. It refers to displacement of a portion of the stomach through the opening in the diaphragm through which the oesophagus passes from the chest to the abdominal cavity. In this disease, a part of the upper wall of the stomach protrudes through the diaphragm at the point where the gullet passes from the chest area to the abdominal area.

The diaphragm is a large dome-shaped muscle dividing the chest form the abdominal cavity. It is the muscle concerned with breathing and it is assisted by the muscles between the ribs during exertion. It has special openings in it to allow for the passage of important blood vessels and for the food channel, the oesophagus. Hiatus hernia occurs at the oesophagus opening.

There are two main types of hiatus hernia, known as 'sliding' type and 'rolling' or para-oesophageal type. In the first type, which is very common, the upper part of the stomach and the cardio-oesophageal junction rise up through the diaphragm by direct herniation through the hiatus. In the second type, which is far less common, a portion of the upper stomach herniates through the hiatus alongside the oesophagus so that cardio-oesophageal junction maintains its normal relationship to the diaphragm.

This disease is quite common after the middle age. It is estimated that about half the people above 60 years of age suffer from it, although most of them may not have any symptoms. Thus well over half of all elderly people have a hiatus hernia or free oesophageal regurgitation. This can cause trouble. It is often difficult to distinguish the chest pain of hiatus hernia from that of coronary artery disease. Both these conditions are so common in old age that they often occur in the same individual, and this should be kept in view before undertaking treatment for one or other of these disorders. The correct diagnosis of hiatus hernia can be arrived at by means of a barium meal x-ray test.

Symptoms

Hiatus hernia is characterised by pain in certain areas. The most common areas are behind the breast bone, at the nipple level and at the lower end of the breast bone. Pain also occurs on the left side of the chest and this is often mistaken for angina. Other areas of pain are the base of the throat, right lower ribs and behind the right shoulder blade. The pain increases when the patient stoops with effort and lies down.

Other symptoms of this disease are heart-burn, especially after a meal, a feeling of fullness and bloatedness, flatulence and discomfort on swallowing. The inflammatory changes often result in occult bleeding and when continued leads to iron deficiency anaemia. In fact, hiatus hernia is probably the main cause of iron deficiency anaemia due to blood loss in elderly patients.

Causes

The chief cause of the mechanical defect associated with hiatus hernia is faulty diet. The consumption of white flour, refined sugar and products made from them such as cakes, pastries, biscuits and white bread as well as preservatives, and flavouring devitalise the system and weaken the muscle tone. As a consequence, the muscles become less resilient, and connective and fibrous tissue suffers through poor nourishment, and thus becomes more prone to decomposition and damage. This ultimately leads to diseases like hiatus hernia.

Drinks like tea, coffee, alcohol also affect the mucous lining of the stomach and irritate the digestive tract. These drinks when taken with meals, encourage fermentation and produce gas. This increases the distension of the stomach, causing pressure against the diaphragm and the oesophageal opening and greatly increasing the risk of herniation. Other causes of hiatus hernia include sedentary occupations, without sensible exercise, overweight resulting form overeating, smoking, shallow breathing and mental and emotional tensions.

Treatment

In the beginning of the treatment, it will be advisable to raise the head end of the bed by placing bricks below the legs of the bed. This will prevent the regurgitation of food during the night. More pillows can also be used for the same purpose.

The next important step towards treating hiatus hernia is relaxation. An important measure in this direction is diaphragmatic breathing. The procedure is as follows: Lie down with both knees bent and feet close to buttocks. Feel relaxed, put both the hands lightly on the abdomen and concentrate the attention on this area. Now breathe in, gently, pushing the abdomen up under the hands at the same time, until no more air can be inhaled. Then relax, breathing out through the mouth with an audible sighing sound and allow the abdominal wall to sink back. The shoulders and chest should remain at rest throughout.

It is important to be able to relax at any time and thereby

prevent building up of physical and mental tensions which may cause actual physical symptoms. The best method for this is to practise shavasana or 'dead body' pose.

The patient of hiatus hernia should observe certain precautions in eating habits. The foremost among these is not to take water with meals, but half an hour before or an hour after a meal. This helps the digestive process considerably and reduces the incident of heart-burn. Drinking water with meals increases the overall weight in the stomach, slows down the digestive process by diluting the digestive juices and this increases the risk of fermentation and gas formation, which distends the stomach and causes discomfort and pain. Another important factor in the treatment of this disease is to take frequent small meals instead of three large ones. Thorough mastication of food is also essential, both to break up the food into small particles and to slow down the rate of intake.

The diet of the patient should consist of seeds, nuts and whole cereal grains, vegetables and fruits, with emphasis on fresh fruits, raw or lightly-cooked vegetables and sprouted seeds. The foods which should be avoided are over-processed foods like white bread, sugar, cakes, biscuits, rice puddings and overcooked vegetables. At least 50 per cent of the diet should consist of fruits and vegetables, and the remaining 50 per cent of protein, carbohydrates and fat.

Raw juices extracted from fresh fruits and vegetables are valuable in hiatus hernia, and the patient should take these juices half an hour before each meal. Carrot juice is especially beneficial as it has a very restorative effect, being rich in Vitamin A and calcium. It is an alkaline food, which soothes the stomach. Tomato juice is also very beneficial. A glassful of fresh tomato juice, mixed with a pinch of salt and pepper, taken early in the morning, will relieve the constant burning sensation in the chest due to hiatus hernia.

The use of rice has been found valuable in hiatus hernia. A thick gruel of rice mixed with a glassful of buttermilk and a well ripe banana taken twice daily is a very nutritious diet in indigestion and burning caused by hiatus hernia.

The hot drinks should always be allowed to cool a little before taking. Extremes in temperature both in food and drink should be avoided. Drinks should not be taken hurriedly. The patient should avoid condiments, pickles, tea, coffee, alcoholic beverages and smoking.

CHAPTER 33

Peptic Ulcer

Peptic ulcer is one of the most common diseases of gastro-intestinal system. It refers to an eroded lesion in the gastric intestinal mucosa. An ulcer may form in any part of the digestive tract which is exposed to acid gastric juice, but is usually found in the stomach and the duodenum. The ulcer in the stomach is known as gastric ulcer and that located in the duodenum is called a duodenal ulcer. Usually, both are grouped together and termed peptic ulcer.

Duodenal ulcers are about 10 times more frequent than gastric ulcers. The incidence of peptic ulcers is four times higher in men than women. Men are more affected by duodenal ulcers whereas women usually get ulcers in the stomach. Both kinds reach a peak in middle age. They, however, remain sufficiently common in old age to cause a lot of trouble. Some peptic ulcers are very chronic one which first develop in middle age but there are many patients who first get ulcer symptom in old age.

Symptoms

The most common symptoms of peptic ulcer are sharp and severe pain and discomfort in the upper central abdomen. The pain is commonly described as burning or gnawing in character. Gastric ulcer pain usually occurs an hour after meals and rarely at night.

Duodenal ulcer pain usually occurs between meals when the stomach is empty and is relieved by food, especially milk. It is often described as hunger pain. As the disease progresses there is distension of the stomach due to excessive flatulence, besides mental tension, insomnia and gradual weakening of the body. It may also cause constipation with occasional blood in the stools.

A really severe peptic ulcer can lead to serious complications like haemorrhage, perforation or obstruction of the orifice through which the food passes from the stomach to the intestine. Unless treated in time, it can lead to massive bleeding and shock, or even death.

Peptic ulcers in old age may be present in a variety of ways. Some elderly patients may suffer from weight loss, general debility, anaemia or painless vomiting. The symptom of pain is often absent in old age because the elderly may have a reduced inflammatory response to tissue injury. The most serious complication of peptic ulcer in old age is haemorrhage. When haemorrhage is acute, it may result in death. Chronic haemorrhage may give rise to iron deficiency anaemia.

Causes

Peptic ulcers result from hyperacidity which is a condition caused by an increase in hydrochloric acid in the stomach. This strong acid, secreted by the cells lining the stomach, affects much of the break-down of food. It can be potentially dangerous and, under certain circumstances, it may eat its way through the lining of the stomach or duodenum producing, first, irritation of the stomach wall, and eventually an ulcer.

Dietetic indiscretion, like overeating, taking of heavy meals or highly spiced foods, coffee, alcohol and smoking are the main factors contributing to this condition. Alcohol is a very powerful acid producer and has a burning effect on the stomach lining. Coffee also increases the production of acid especially when it is taken black. The ingestion of certain drugs, particularly aspirin, food poisoning, infections like influenza and septicaemia and gout may also cause ulcers.

Emotional stress or nervous tension also plays a major role in the formation of ulcers. The stomach is a highly sensitive organ and nervous activity can slow down or speed up digestion. Those given to excessive worry, anger, tension, jealousy and hurry are thus more prone to suffer from ulcers than those who are easy-going and relaxed. Ulcer patients are usually highly strung, irritable and ambitious people who live very active lives. They generally take on many things at one time and worry about the results of their various projects.

Treatment

Persons who treat themselves with antacids may do themselves more harm than good. Though they may get initial relief because the tablet neutralises the acid, the stomach responds by producing even more acid because the basic cause of the hyperacidity has not been dealt with. Ulcers can be best treated by natural methods.

Diet is of utmost importance in the treatment of ulcer. The diet should be so arranged as to provide adequate nutrition to afford rest to the disturbed organs to maintain continuous neutralisation of the gastric acid, to inhibit the production of acid and to reduce mechanical and chemical irritation.

Milk, cream, butter, fruits and fresh, raw and boiled vegetables and natural foods are the best diet for an ulcer patient. The fruits recommended are banana, mango, musk melon and dates. Such a diet will progressively reduce the acidity in the stomach. A low-salt diet can greatly help in curing hyperacidity and ulcers.

The use of banana and plantain is considered highly beneficial in the treatment of peptic ulcer. These fruits are antiulcerogenic and have long been used in folk medicine to treat ulcers. They are said to contain an unidentified compound called, perhaps jokingly,

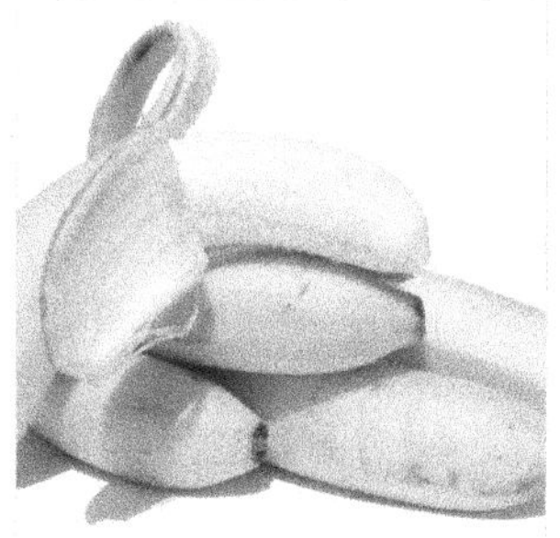

Vitamin U (against ulcers). According to British pharmacist Dr. Ralph Best of the University of Aston in Birmingham, bananas stimulate proliferation of cells and mucus that form a stronger barrier between the stomach lining and corrosive acid. Plantains should, however, be cooked before eating because they are too hard and tough to eat raw. Green plantains are considered a more potent medicine for healing ulcers than ripe ones.

Cabbage is another useful remedy for peptic ulcers. It contains antiulcer drugs. In a research study, Dr. Garnett Chenery, a professor of medicine at Stanford University School of Medicine in the 1950s, demonstrated that just 850 ml of fresh cabbage juice every day relieved pain and healed both gastric and duodenal ulcers better and faster than standard treatments did. In a test of 55 patients who drank cabbage juice, 95 per cent felt better within two to five days. X-rays and gastroscopy revealed a rapid healing of gastric ulcers in only one-quarter of the average time. The duodenal ulcers of patients fed cabbage also healed in one-third the usual time. Cabbage can also be boiled in water and this water taken twice daily after cooling.

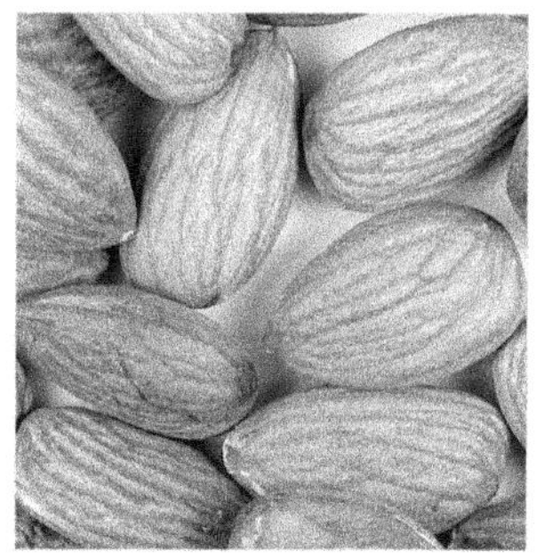

Almond milk made from blanched almonds in a blender is also beneficial in the treatment of ulcer. It binds the excess of acid in the stomach and supplies high-quality protein. Raw goat's milk is also highly beneficial. It actually helps to heal peptic ulcer.

Raw fruits and vegetables should be avoided for a few weeks, as many of these are especially irritating. Potatoes and squashes are, however, well-tolerated. All sour fruits should be avoided, especially citrus fruits.

Certain foods do not agree in cases of gastric complaints and should be eliminated. These include fried and greasy foods which are always difficult to digest; fresh foods which require a high amount of acid in the stomach for their digestion and acid causes more pain and flatulence in the sensitive stomach; condiments, preserves and sugar which are stomach irritants; and tea, coffee, tobacco and alcohol which create an acidic reaction in the stomach. The healing capacity and vitality of the body will increase if these harmful and unsuitable foods are avoided.

How rapidly the ulcer heals will largely depend on the correct assortment of essential amino acids and sufficient ascorbic acid. Iron absorption depends on an acid medium and is facilitated by the presence of ascorbic acid. The neutralisation of stomach acid, therefore, interferes with iron absorption. Several studies have shown that Vitamin E and A, especially taken together, have not only a protective effect against development of ulcers caused by stress, but also a curative effect on existing ulcers.

The observance of certain rules by an ulcer patient with regard to eating habits are essential. He should never eat when tired or emotionally upset, nor when he is not hungry even if it is mealtime, nor when his mouth is dry. He should chew every morsel thoroughly. He should eat only natural foods and take food in as dry a form as possible. Meals must be small and frequent. All foods and drinks which are either too hot or too cold should be avoided.

The patient should drink eight to 10 glasses of water every day. However, he should not drink water during or with meals, but only half an hour before or one hour after he has eaten.

In case of haemorrhage in the stomach, a rectal enema should be administered four times daily with the water temperature at 110° to 115°. In case of abdominal or stomach pain, hot packs should be placed on the abdomen with water temperature at 120°F. Hot pack should also be placed between the shoulder blades.

Daily massage and deep breathing exercises also help. Above all, the patient must try to rid himself of his worries and stay cheerful. He should also cultivate regularity in his habits — be it work, exercise or rest.

CHAPTER 34

Constipation

Constipation is a common disturbance of the digestive tract. In this condition, the bowels do not move regularly, or are not completely emptied when they move.

Constipation is a common problem in the elderly. This is evident from studies which indicate that people in the age group of over 60 years use more laxatives than any other age group. And all attempts to persuade them to discontinue their use do not succeed. As age advances, the body burns up energy slowly and digestive processes are affected. The bowel movements also become sluggish. This leads to constipation.

Constipation is the chief cause of many diseases as such a condition produces toxins which find their way into the bloodstream and are carried to all parts of the body. This results in weakening of the vital organs and lowering of the resistance of the entire system. Appendicitis, rheumatism, arthritis, high blood pressure, cataract and cancer are only a few of the diseases in which chronic constipation is an important predisposing factor.

A number of motions required for normal health varies from person to person. Most people have one motion a day, some have two a day, while others have one every other day. However, for comfort and health, at least one clear bowel movement a day is essential and considered normal.

Symptoms

The most common symptoms of constipation are infrequency, irregularity or difficulty of elimination due to hard faecal matter. Among the other symptoms are coated tongue, foul breath, loss of appetite, headache, dizziness, dark circles under the eyes, depression, nausea, pimples on the face, ulcers in the mouth, constant fullness in the abdomen, diarrhoea alternating with constipation, varicose veins, pain in the lumber region, acidity, heart-burn and insomnia.

Causes

The most important causes for chronic constipation are wrong dietary and faulty style of living. All foods in their natural state contain a good percentage of 'roughage' which is most essential in preserving natural balance of foods and also in helping peristalsis — the natural rhythmic action by means of which the food is passed down the alimentary canal. Much of the food we eat today is very deficient in natural bulk or roughage and this results in chronic constipation.

Intake of refined and rich foods lacking in vitamins and minerals, insufficient intake of water, consumption of meat in large quantities, excessive use of strong tea and coffee, insufficient chewing, overeating and wrong combination of foods, irregular habits of eating and drinking may all contribute to poor bowel function. Other causes include faulty and irregular habit of defecation, frequent use of purgatives, weakness of abdominal muscles due to sedentary habits, lack of physical activity and emotional stress and strain.

Elderly persons may suffer from constipation due to a variety of factors. It has been said that the movement of the intestines is directly proportional to the movement of the legs. Elderly people have limited physical activity because of stiff joints, arthritis or other physical and mental illnesses. With advancing age, appetite also is reduced. Falling teeth contribute to reduced food intake which adds to the problem of constipation. Elderly people also tend to stop eating on the presumption that unless the already eaten food is digested and evacuated, they should not eat further. This compounds the problem of constipation. The use of drugs by the elderly for treating certain ailments commonly prevalent in them like insominia, high blood pressure. Diabetes and cough can also lead to constipation in old age.

Treatment

The purgatives and laxatives give only temporary relief. They unnecessarily irritate the stomach and intestines, weakening the colon. Laxative abuse may also lead to low blood potassium and long term chronic ill health. The natural way to treat constipation is to give up all artificial aids. The observance of regular hours for meals, elimination and sleep, a balanced diet, sufficient exercise, and a high standard of general health with good muscular tone are essential in the treatment of constipation.

The most important factor in curing constipation is natural and simple diet. This should consist of unrefined foods such as whole grain cereals, bran, honey, molasses and lentils; green and leafy vegetables, especially spinach, french beans, tomatoes, lettuce, onion, cabbage, cauliflower, brussels sprouts, celery, turnip, pumpkin, peas, beets, asparagus, carrot, fresh fruits, especially pears, grapes, figs, papaya, mangoes, guava and oranges; dry fruits such as figs, raisins, apricots and dates; milk products in the form of butter, ghee and cream.

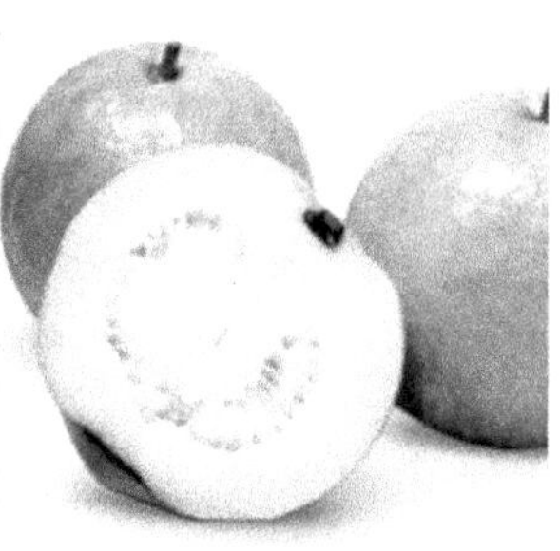

The diet alone is not enough. Food should be properly chewed — each morsel for at least 15 times. Hurried meals and meals at odd times should be avoided. Sugar and sugary foods should be strictly avoided because sugar steals B Vitamins from the body, without which the intestines cannot function normally. Foods which constipate are all products made of white flour, pastries, biscuits, cheese, fresh foods, preserves, white sugar and hard boiled eggs.

Regular drinking of water is beneficial not only for constipation but also for cleaning the system, diluting the blood, and washing out poisons. Normally about eight glasses of water should be taken daily as it is essential for digesting and dissolving food nutrients so that they can be absorbed and utilised by the body. Water should, however, not be taken with meals as it dilutes the gastric juices essential for proper digestion. Water should be taken either half an hour before or an hour after meals.

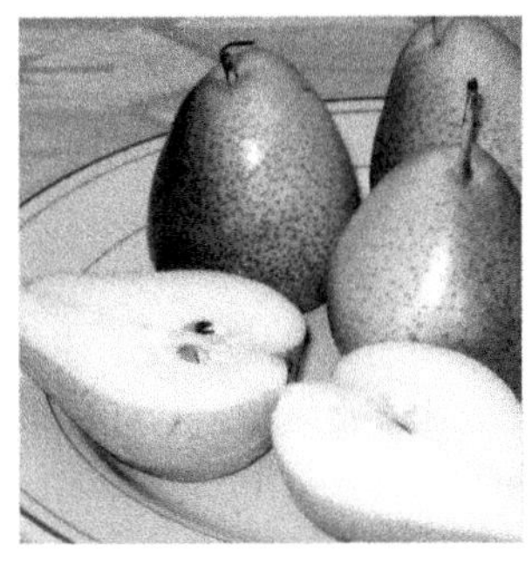

Generally, all fruits, except banana and jack fruit, are beneficial in the treatment of constipation. Certain fruits are, however, more effective. Pears are regarded as one of the best laxative fruits. Those suffering from chronic constipation should adopt an exclusive diet of this fruit or its juice for a few days, but in ordinary cases, a medium-sized pear taken after the dinner or with breakfast will have the desired effect. The same is true of guava which, when eaten with seeds, gives roughage to the diet and helps in the normal evacuation of the bowels.

Grapes have proved highly beneficial in overcoming constipation. The combination of the properties of the cellulose, sugar and organic acid in grapes make them a laxative food. Their field of action is not limited to clearing the bowels only. They also tone up the stomach and intestines and relieve the most chronic constipation. One should take at least 350 grams of grapes daily to achieve the desired results. When fresh grapes are not available, raisins soaked in water can be used. Raisins should be soaked in a tumblerful of drinking water for 24 to 48 hours. This would swell them to the original size of the grapes. These raisins should be eaten early in the morning. The water in which raisins are soaked should also be drunk along with the soaked raisins.

Drinking hot water with sour lime juice and half a tea spoon of salt is also an effective remedy for constipation. Drinking water which has been kept overnight in copper vessel, first thing in the morning will bring good results. Linseed is extremely useful in difficult cases of constipation. A teaspoon of linseeds, swallowed with water before each meal, provides both bulk and lubrication.

In all ordinary cases of constipation, an exclusive fruit diet for about seven days would be the best way to begin the treatment. For long-standing and stubborn cases, it would be advisable to have a short fast for four or five days. This will drive out the packed contents of the bowels, eliminate toxins and purify the blood stream. The weak patients may take orange juice during the period of fasting. After the all-fruit diet or the short fast, as the case may be, the patient should gradually embark upon a balanced diet comprising adequate raw foods, ripe fruits and whole grain cereals. In some cases, further short periods or short fasts may be necessary at intervals of two months or so depending on the progress being made. The bowels should be cleansed daily through a warm water enema for a few days at the commencement of the treatment.

A cold friction bath taken daily in the morning can help cure constipation. An alternate hot and cold hip bath, taken before retiring to bed, is also beneficial. Fresh air, outdoor games, walking, swimming, gardening and other exercises play an important role in strengthening and activating the muscles, and thereby prevent constipation.

Certain yogic asanas also help to bring relief from constipation as they strengthen the abdominal and pelvic muscles and stimulate the peristalic action of the bowels. These asanas are bhujangasana, shalabhasana, yogamudra, dhanurasana and paschimotanasana.

CHAPTER 35

Diarrhoea

Diarrhoea refers to the frequent passage of loose or watery unformed stools. As a rough guide, it can be said that three or four loose or watery stools a day can be considered as diarrhoea. The disease may be acute or chronic.

Commonly known as "Loose motion," diarrhoea is perhaps the most common disease in India, both in the young and elderly. It can pose a great threat to those elderly people who are frail and weak. A lot of difficulties are experienced in diagnosing the disease in the elderly.

The intestine normally gets more than 10 litres of liquid per day which comes from the diet and from secretion of the stomach, liver, pancreas and intestines. In the case of diarrhoea, water is either not absorbed or is secreted in excess by the organs of the body. It is then sent to the colon where water holding capacity is limited. Thus the urge to defecate comes quite often.

Causes

The chief causes of diarrhoea are overeating or eating of wrong foods, putrefaction in intestinal tract, fermentation caused by incomplete carbohydrate digestion and nervous irritability. Other causes include parasites, germs, virus, bacteria or a poison which has entered into the body through food, water or air, allergies to certain substances or even common foods such as milk, wheat, eggs and sea foods and emotional strain or stress.

Diarrhoea may be a prominent feature of organic diseases affecting the small or large intestine such as the sprue syndrome, malignant disease and ulcerative colitis. It may also result from operations on the gastrointestinal tract. Diarrhoea may alternate with constipation. This may result from the irritation of the mucous membrane by impacted hard faeces.

Diarrhoea in the elderly may be caused by several factors. Acute diarrhoea often results from dietary indiscretion, particularly from excessive consumption of laxative foods. Liberal use of purgatives and excessive self-medication with laxatives may cause long-standing diarrhoea. Diarrhoea in the elderly may also result as a side effect of certain drugs for treating other diseases such as antibiotics. The use of antibiotics can lead to destruction of the friendly bacteria in intestines along with pathogenic bacteria at which the antibiotic treatment was aimed at.

Complications

Diarrhoea for prolonged periods can lead to certain complications. These may include weakness due to loss of vitamins like A, D, E and K and other nutrients as food is rushed through the body without giving the nutrients a chance of being absorbed, dehydration due to loss of body fluids and washing out of minerals from the body and nervous conditions.

Among the various complications, dehydration poses a serious problem, especially when diarrhoea is accompanied by vomiting. It can even be fatal if unchecked. Dehydration is characterised by hot, dry skin over the abdomen, sunken eyes, dry mouth, intense thirst and reduced flow of urine. This can usually be prevented, if the patient suffering from diarrhoea, with or without vomiting, is given plenty of liquids. The patient should be given about 150-200 ml. of fluid every hour from 6 a.m. to 10 p.m.

Treatment

No drugs should be taken to control diarrhoea as it has been found that anti-diarrhoeal drugs and binding mixture may temporarily relieve the symptoms, but do not really help to cure the disease. Rather they hamper the bowel's protective function to rid the body of its harmful contents.

In severe cases of diarrhoea, it is advisable to observe a complete fast for two days to provide rest for the gastrointestinal tract. Hot water only may be taken during the period to compensate for the loss of fluids. Juices of fruits may be taken after the acute symptoms are over. After condition improves, meals can be enlarged gradually to include cooked vegetables, whole rice, soured milks. Raw foods should be taken only after the patient completely recovers.

An effective remedy for diarrhoea is the use of buttermilk. It is the residual milk left after the fat has been removed from yoghurt by churning. It helps overcome harmful intestinal flora and re-establish the benign or friendly flora. The acid in the buttermilk also fghts germs and bacteria. It may be mixed with a pinch of salt three or four times a day for controlling diarrhoea.

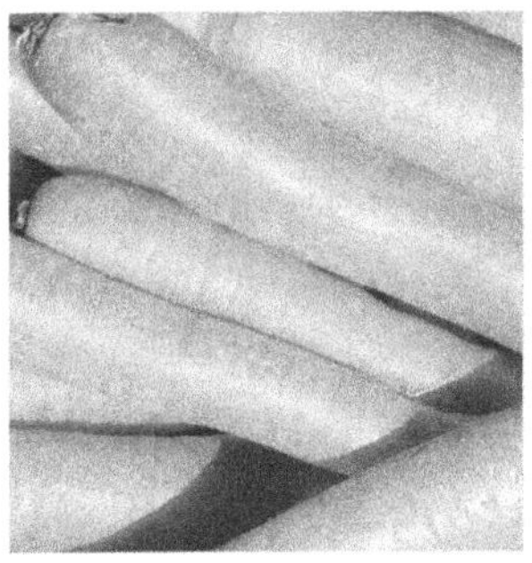

Carrot soup is another effective home remedy for diarrhoea. It supplies water to combat dehydration, replenishes sodium, potassium, phosphorus, calcium, sulphur and magnesium, supplies pectin and coats the intestine to allay inflammation. It checks the growth of harmful intestinal bacteria and prevents vomitting. Half a kg. of carrot may be cooked in 150 ml. of water until it is soft. The pulp should be strained and boiled water added to make a litre. Three-quarter tablespoon of salt may be mixed. This soup should be given in small amounts to the patient every half an hour.

The pomegranate has proved beneficial in the treatment of diarrhoea because of its astringent properties. If the patient develops weakness due to profuse and continuous purging, he should be given repeatedly about 50 ml. of pomegranate juice to drink. This will control the diarrhoea.

Turmeric has proved another effective home remedy for diarrhoea. It is a very useful intestinal antiseptic. It is also a gastric stimulant and a tonic. Turmeric rhizome, its juice or dry powder are all very helpful in curing chronic diarrhoea. In the form of dry powder, it may be taken in buttermilk or plain water.

In case of diarrhoea caused by indigestion, dry or fresh ginger is very useful. A piece of dry ginger is powdered along with a crystal of rock salt. A quarter teaspoon of this powder should be taken with a small piece of jaggery. It will bring quick relief as ginger, being carminative, aids digestion by stimulating the gastrointestinal tract.

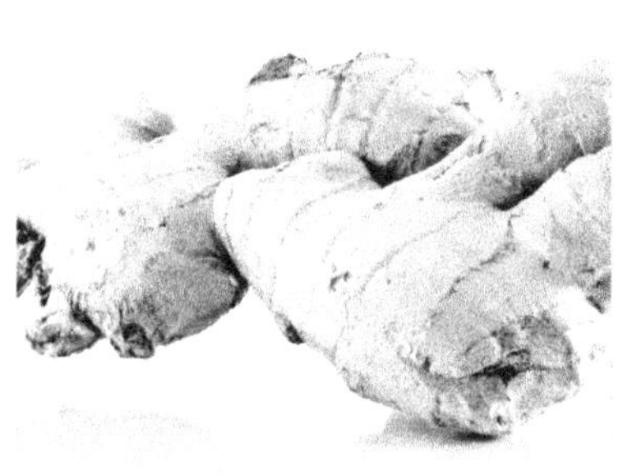

Starchy liquids such as arrowroot water, barley water, rice gruel and coconut water are beneficial in the treatment of diarrhoea. They not only replace the fluid lost but also bind the stools. Other home remedies include bananas and garlic. Bananas contain pectin and encourage the growth of beneficial bacteria. Garlic is a powerful, effective and harmless antibiotic. It aids digestion and routs parasites.

The best water treatments for diarrhoea are the abdominal compress (at 60°F) renewed every 15 to 20 minutes and cold hip bath (40°-50°F). If the patient is in pain, abdominal fomentations for 15 minutes should be administered every two hours. The procedure for these treatments are given in the Appendix.

CHAPTER 36

Diverticulosis

Diverticulosis is a condition of the colon, in which the muscular wall gives way in places and allows the mucous membrane lining the large intestine to form pouches. These pouches are known as diverticula, a name which comes from the word "diverted." They become lodging places for decaying particles of food or faecal matter. The disease by itself is of no consequence. Sometimes, however, diverticula become inflamed, as they do not have muscles in their walls and cannot empty themselves. This condition is known as diverticulitis. The disease is usually established by means of x-rays.

Diverticulosis usually occurs in the middle and later years. The incidence of this disease rises with age and the post-mortem studies have shown that above 50 per cent of older persons suffer from it.

Symptoms

The main symptoms of diverticulitis are pain in the left lower side of the abdomen, diarrhoea or constipation or alteration of the two, and bleeding. Attacks may recur over a long time.

Severe complications may arise from the tendency of obstructed diverticula to perforate and thus give rise to pericolic abcess, peritonitis or fistula to bladder, vagina or other parts of the guts.

Inflammatory masses may form and may result in obstructive symptoms which closely resemble carcinoma of the colon. Such complications may require surgical treatment.

Persons with diverticulosis frequently develop anaemia. The bacteria in the diverticula, caused by stagnant food and faecal matter, appear to grab all the Vitamin B, folic acid from the food and prevent it from reaching the blood. This condition is corrected when these putrefactive bacteria are destroyed by a generous intake of yoghurt or acidophilus milk, provided the diet contains folic acid. The patient may also develop other intestinal and general problems due to the increase of toxins generated by this condition.

Causes

The prime cause of diverticulosis or diverticulitis is low-residue diet of highly refined foods. The disease is rare in primitive tribes, who consume high-roughage diet. It is thus, primarily a deficiency disease caused by deficiency of 'high-residue' foods like whole, unrefined, natural and bulky foods.

Another cause of this disease is severe mental tension. When tension is great, gas cannot be expelled normally and is forced against the intestinal walls. This may sometimes lead to the formation of diverticula and ultimately result in diverticulosis or diverticulitis.

Treatment

Modern medical system in most cases prescribes surgery to remove the diverticula. But the surgical removal of old diverticula does not prevent the formation of new ones. The best way to treat the disease is through natural methods. The treatment should aim at improving digestion, decreasing gas formation, building stronger intestinal walls to resist the formation of diverticula and relieving stress to avoid tension building up in the body.

Diet plays an important role in this treatment. The emphasis should be on high roughage diet consisting of seeds, nuts and whole grains, vegetables and fruits. Seeds may be consumed in the sprouted form. Cooked cereals like millet, brown rice and oats are beneficial. Soured milks like yoghurt and buttermilk, potatoes and flax seeds should be taken daily in adequate quantities.

The patient should take small, frequent meals, rather than few large ones. He should avoid refined and processed foods, tea, coffee, condiments, pickles and animal foods.

If the disease is accompanied by constipation, all measures should be adopted for its eradication through natural methods. Purgatives should not be used. If constipation occurs despite the patient adhering to the diet of natural foods, warm water enema should be used to cleanse the bowels. If the patient is overweight, he should take a diet of natural foods aimed at reducing the weight.

The use of bran is considered highly beneficial in the treatment of diverticulosis or diverticulitis. Unprocessed wheat bran has five times the fibre of ordinary whole wheat The quantity of bran to be used varies from one table spoon daily to three table spoons three times a day, depending on the severity of the disease. Most of the patients, however, need two spoons of bran three times a day, to render the stools soft and easy to pass. The quantity can be increased, if necessary, after two weeks until the patient can move his bowels once or twice a day without straining. As it is difficult to eat just plain bran, it may be sprinkled on cereals, or mixed with porridge, or added to soup or taken with milk or water.

Certain vegetable juices have been found beneficial in the treatment of diverticulosis. These include juice extracted from carrot, beet and green vegetables. The best fruit juices are those extracted from papaya, apple, pineapple and lemon.

The use of vitamins can also help in diverticulosis. Vitamin E is a well-known muscle strengthener and should be used liberally by the patient. Vitamins of B group are needed, not only to provide the folic acid but to prevent stress and strengthen nerves. Vitamin

C can help greatly in removing toxic matter from the body. Minerals are also needed in diverticulosis, potassium, manganese, calcium and magnesium, all can help strengthen muscular and nervous systems.

Diverticulosis and diverticulitis can be treated successfully through natural methods as outlined above. Surgery may be resorted to in rare cases, where there is severe obstruction, perforation or abscess formation or where there is severe involvement of the intestine.

CHAPTER 37

Colitis

Colitis is an inflammation of the colon or large intestine. There are two types of colitis: mucus and ulcerative. Mucus colitis is a common disorder of the large bowel, producing discomfort and irregular bowel habits. Chronic ulcerative colitis is a severe prolonged inflammation of the colon or large bowel in which ulcers form on the walls of the colon resulting in the passing of bloody stools with pus and mucus.

Both forms of colitis are the results of prolonged irritation of the delicate membrane which lines the walls of the colon. About 25 per cent of all cases of ulcerative colitis occur in the elderly. The disease may also appear for the first time in old age.

Normally, it is the function of the colon to store waste material until most of the fluids have been removed to enable well-formed soft stools, consisting of non-absorbable food materials to be passed. Persons who suffer from an irritable colon have irregular and erratic contractions which are specially noticeable on the left side.

Symptoms

Chronic ulcerative colitis usually begins in the lower part of the bowels and spreads upwards. The first symptom of the trouble is an increased urgency to move the bowel, followed by cramping pains in the abdomen and bloody mucus in the stools. As the disease spreads upwards, the stools become watery and more frequent and are characterised by rectal straining. All the loss of blood and fluid from the bowels results in weakness, fever, nausea, vomiting, loss of apetite and anaemia.

The patient may develop a bloated feeling because the gas is not absorbed or expelled normally. Some patients suffer from constipation alternating with periods of loose bowel movements. Still others may suffer from persistent diarrhoea for years together. The patient is usually malnourished and may be severely underweight. He may suffer form frequent insomnia.

The most prominent symptom of ulcerative colitis in the elderly is diarrhoea which may be associated with faecal incontinence. This may be associated with lower abdominal pain, tenesmus and urgency of micturition. Haemorrhage is less common in the elderly than in younger patients. It may be difficult to diagnose perforation with acute peritonitis in the elderly because of the absence of pain. The elderly patient may suffer from acute brain failure and a toxic state may appear.

Ulcerative colitis in its severe form may lead to nutritional problems. The improper assimilation of the ingested foods, due to inflammatory conditions, may cause deficiency diseases. This may gradually result in nervous irritability, exhaustion and depression. In very severe cases, the patient may even develop suicidal tendencies.

Causes

The main cause of colitis is chronic constipation and the use of laxatives and purgatives. Constipation causes an accumulation of the hard faecal matter which is never properly evacuated. The frequent use of saline laxatives like Epsom salt, liver salts and fruit salts and antacid powders and soda bicarb for digestive troubles, retard the normal secretion of hydrochloric acid, which may result in colitis. The use of mineral oil laxatives like paraffin oil neutralises Vitamin A and the other fat-soluble vitamins, the deficiency of which can cause colitis.

Often, colitis is caused by poorly-digested roughage, especially of cereals and carbohydrates, which causes bowel irritation. It may also result from an allergic sensitivity to certain foods, especially milk, wheat and eggs. Often, the intake of antibiotics may upset the bacterial flora in the intestines and interfere with proper digestion.

Severe stress may also produce ulcerative colitis. During any form of severe stress, outpouring of adrenal hormones causes such destruction of body protein that at times parts of the walls lining the intestines are literally eaten away. Such stress also depletes the body of pantothenic acid. Experiments on animals have shown that they can develop ulcerative colitis when they are kept on diets deficient in pantothenic acid.

Treatment

The usual treatment of colitis with suppressive drugs is based on the assumption that colitis is due to germ infection, which it is not. The suppressive drugs drive back into the system the toxic matter in the colon which nature is endeavoring to eliminate in the form of mucus. They suppress the symptoms temporarily, without removing the cause. In such cases, the symptoms recur and colitis becomes chronic. Plain warm water or warm water with a little olive oil used as washout is the only method of softening and removing the accumulations of hardened matter sticking to the walls of the colon.

Diet plays an important part in the treatment of colitis. It is advisable to observe a juice fast for five days or so in most cases of colitis. The juices may be diluted with a little boiled water. Papaya juice, raw cabbage and carrot juices are especially beneficial. Citrus juices should be avoided. The bowels should be cleansed daily with a warm water enema.

After the juice fast, the patient should gradually adopt a diet of small, frequent meals of soft cooked or steamed vegetables, rice, dalia (coarsely broken wheat) and well-ripened fruits like banana, papaya, yoghurt and home-made cottage cheese. Sprouted seeds and grains, whole wheat bread and raw vegetables may be added gradually to this diet after about 10 days. Tender coconut water is highly beneficial as it is soothing to the soft mucosa of the colon. Cooked apple also aids the healing of ulcerative conditions because of its ample concentration of iron and phosphorus. All foods must be eaten slowly and chewed thoroughly.

Foods which should be excluded from the diet are white sugar, white bread and white flour products, highly seasoned foods, highly salted foods, strong tea, coffee and alcoholic beverages and foods cooked in aluminum pans.

Vitamins and proteins are vital in the prevention and treatment of colitis. The colon is lined with mucous membrane, which requires, Vitamin A for its healthy maintenance. When the mucous surface of the colon is deprived of this vitamin, it gradually deteriorates and becomes sensitive, spongy, and ulcerated. During illness, the need for Vitamin A is greatly increased because the stored supply is rapidly exhausted. Vitamins of the B group are lacking in the modern dietary of refined and processed foods. As a result, stomach disorders arise which have an adverse effect upon the colon. Vitamin C is required for strengthening the connective tissue in which the cells are embedded, and also the walls of blood vessels. Calcium is of value too, in relieving the spasms in the intestines which occur in some forms of colitis.

The patient should also take protein-rich foods, as otherwise the muscular walls and ligaments will weaken and the colon will be inadequately supported. As a consequence, food will remain undigested, waste products will accumulate in the colon, and the subsequent use of laxatives to remove them will cause irritation and lead to colitis.

Ripe bananas are ideal in the treatment of ulcerative colitis, being bland, smooth, easily digested and slightly laxative. They relieve acute symptoms and promote the healing process.

An effective remedy for ulcerative colitis is the use of buttermilk. It is the residual milk left after the fat has been removed from yoghurt by churning. Buttermilk enema twice a week is also soothing and helps in re-installing a healthy flora in the colon.

Drumstick (sanjana) alleviates colitis. A teaspoon of fresh leaf juice, mixed with an equal quantity of honey and a glass of tender coconut water, is given two or three times daily as a herbal medicine.

Rice has a very low fibre content, and is, therefore, extremely soothing in colitis. A thick gruel of rice mixed with a glass of buttermilk and a ripe banana, given twice a day, forms a very nutritious, well-balanced diet in this disease.

The juice of wheat-grass (a grass which grows after sowing wheat grains in the earth) used as an enema, helps detoxify the walls of the colon. The general procedure is to first give an enema with lukewarm water. After waiting for twenty minutes, 90-120 ml of wheat-grass juice enema is given. This should be retained for 15 minutes. This enema is very helpful in disorders associated with colitis. Wheat-grass can be grown at home in earthen pots if it is not available through dealers.

The patient should have a bowel movement at the same time each day and spend 10 to 15 minutes in the endeavour. Straining at stools should be avoided. Drinking two glasses of water first thing in the morning will stimulate a normal movement. An enema may be used if no bowel movement occurs.

Complete bed rest and plenty of liquids are very important. The patient should eliminate all causes of tension, adjust to his disability and face his discomfort with patience.

CHAPTER 38

Piles

Piles or Haemorrhoids are among the most common ailments today, especially in the Western world. They are varicose and often inflamed condition of the veins inside or just outside the rectum. In external piles, there is a lot of pain but not much bleeding. In the case of internal piles, there is discharge of dark blood.

Nearly 40 per cent of people suffer from piles at some stage of their lives. Elderly people form the largest segment of those suffering from this disease. However, many of them do not seek medical advice mainly either due to their shyness or due to relatively painless nature of the disease. It is essential to treat piles in the initial stage to avoid future complications.

Piles are classified from mild to severe depending on the degree of prolapse, that is, how much they protrude from the anus. In some cases, the veins burst and this results in what is known as bleeding piles.

Symptoms

Pain at passing stools, slight bleeding in the case of internal trouble, and a feeling of soreness and irritation after passing a stool are the usual symptoms of piles. The patient cannot sit comfortably due to itching, discomfort and pain in the rectal region.

Certain complication may arise in case piles are untreated or if they are not treated properly. Profuse bleeding may lead to anemia, causing weakness, tiredness and lethargy. Sometimes piles which come out of the anal opening cannot go back due to spasm at the anal opening. This may lead to clotting of blood, giving rise to sudden swelling and pain. In advanced degree of piles, ulceration may develop due to friction, and cause bleeding. Sometimes, many germs, which contaminate the anal region, may infect already eroded piles, and this may lead to pus formation.

Causes

The primary cause of piles is chronic constipation and other bowel disorders. The pressure applied to pass a stool to evacuate constipated bowels and the congestion caused by constipation ultimately lead to piles. The use of purgatives to relieve constipation, by their irritating and weakening effect on the lining of the rectum, also result in enlargement and inflammation of veins and bleeding of the mucous lining. Piles are more common during pregnancy and in condition affecting the liver and upper bowel.

Prolonged periods of standing or sitting, strenuous work, obesity and general weakness of the tissues of the body are the other contributory causes of piles.

Mental tension is also one of the main causes of haemorrhoids. Persons who are always in a hurry often strain while passing stools. They rush through defecation instead of making it a relaxed affair. The pressure thus exerted by the anal muscles affect the surrounding tissues. The extra rectal pressure and resultant congestion of veins ultimately lead to haemorrhoids. There is probably a hereditary factor also involved in the development of piles.

Treatment

There is no local treatment to cure piles. The treatment of the basic cause, namely, chronic constipation, is the only way to get rid of the trouble. To begin with, the whole digestive tract must be given a complete rest for a few days and the intestines thoroughly cleansed. For this purpose, the patient should adopt an all-fruit diet for at least five days. He should have three meals a day of fresh juicy fruits such as grapes, apple, pear, peach, orange, pineapple and melon. For drinks, unsweetened lemon water or plain water either hot or cold may be taken.

In long-standing and stubborn cases, it will be advisable to have a short fast for four or five days before adopting an all-fruit diet. When on short fast, the patient may have the juice of an orange in a glass of warm water. An enema with lukewarm water should be taken daily in the morning while fasting. This will cleanse the bowels and give much needed rest to the rectal tissues.

After the all-fruit diet, the patient may adopt a diet of natural foods aimed at securing soft stools. The diet should be low in fat and should not contain more than 50 grams of fat. Foods which contain less fat are skimmed milk, buttermilk, curd and cottage cheese made from skimmed milk; all vegetables except cabbage, onions, dried beans and peas; cooked and dried cereals, whole wheat chapattis and fruits and fruit juices.

The ideal diet for the patient with piles should consist of fruits like papaya, musk melon, apple and pear; green vegetables, particularly spinach and radish, wheat, porridge, whole meal cereals and milk. Lentils and daals should be avoided, as they constipate the bowels. The patient should also abstain from meat, fish, eggs, cheese, white sugar, sweets, rice, all fried foods,

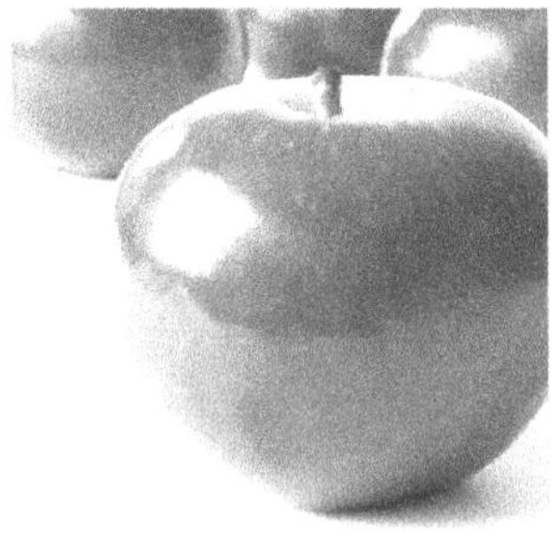

all white flour products, tea and coffee. Dry fruits, such as figs and raisins and coconuts should form part of the diet.

Foods rich in Vitamin C, bioflavonoids and Vitamin E are essential in the treatment of haemorrhoids. Such foods include fresh raw vegetables and fruits, especially cabbage, citrus fruits, whole grains, seeds and nuts. Vitamin B6 also relieves this disease. Piles have been produced in volunteers deficient in Vitamin B6 and corrected when this vitamin was given. The patient with piles should supplement his diet with 10 mg. of B6 after each meal.

The most important food remedy for piles is dry figs. Three or four figs should be soaked overnight in water after cleaning them thoroughly in hot water. They should be taken first thing in the morning along with the water in which they were soaked. They should also be taken in the evening in similar manner. This treatment should be continued for three or four weeks. The tiny seeds of the fruit possess an excellent quality of stimulating peristaltic movements of intestines. This facilitates easy evacuation of faeces and keeps the alimentary canal clean. The pressure on the anus having thus been relieved, the haemorrhoids also get contracted.

The mango seeds are valuable in bleeding piles. The seeds should be collected during the mango season, dried in the shade and powdered and kept stored for use as medicine. This powder should be given in doses of about one and a half gram to two grams with or without honey twice daily.

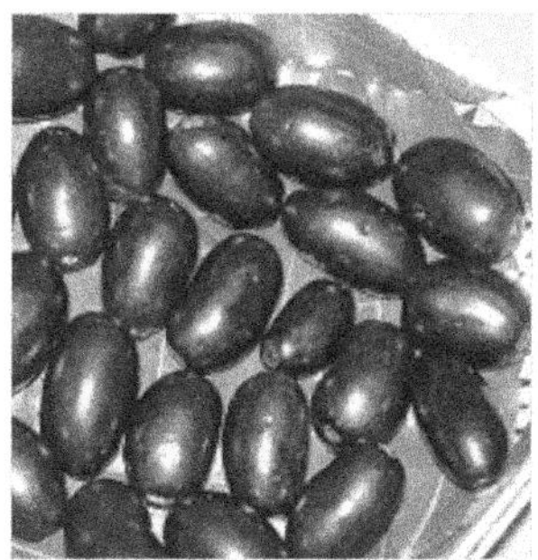

The jambul fruit is another effective food remedy for bleeding piles. The fruit should be taken with salt every morning for two or three months in its season. The use of the fruit in this manner in every season will effect radical cure and save the user from bleeding piles for entire life.

White radish is valuable in piles. Grated radish mixed with honey may be taken in treating this condition. It can also be taken in the form of juice mixed with a pinch of salt. It should be given in doses of 60 to 90 ml. morning and evening. White radish well ground into a paste in milk can also be beneficially applied over inflamed pile masses to relieve pain and swelling.

The patient should drink at least eight to ten glasses of water a day. He should avoid straining to pass stool. Cold water treatment helps the veins to shrink and tones up their walls. The treatment is done by sitting in a tub filled with cold water for two minutes with knees drawn up to your chin. The water level should cover the hips. This should be done twice a day. Other water treatments beneficial in curing piles include cold perineal douche and cold compress applied to the rectal area for an hour before bedtime. Personal hygiene is also important. The area around the anal opening should be washed with soap and warm water and dried with a soft towel.

Exercise plays an important corrective role in this condition. Movements which exercise the abdominal muscles will improve circulation in the rectal region and relieve congestion. Outdoor exercises such as walking and swimming are excellent methods of building up general health. The yogic kriyas like jalneti and vamandhouti and asnas such as sarvangasana, vipritakarani and halasana are also useful. Sarvangasana is especially beneficial as it drains stagnant blood from the anus.

CHAPTER 39

Cirrhosis of the Liver

The liver is one of the most important organs in the body. It serves as a combination of manufacturing plant, chemical laboratory and storehouse of nutrients. It produces many vital elements and pours them into the blood stream, or stores until needed. Some of its functions are the production and storage of substances essential to the manufacture of red blood cells, the elimination of poisons and protein and the regulation of the numerous by-products of protein metabolism, the storage of sugar, the storage and utilisation of fats, the control of cholesterol metabolism, and the production of bile acids, bile salts, and substances important for blood coagulation.

With advancing age, there is some destruction of liver cells. But the body has such an excess of liver tissue that unless there is extreme loss, the liver's functions are not endangered. In normal man, the liver accounts for about 2.5 per cent of body weight at the age of 50. Subsequently, it becomes gradually smaller so that by the age of 90, it represents only 1.6 per cent of body weight. Liver blood flow also decreases in proportion to declining liver volume.

Cirrhosis of the liver is one of the most serious diseases of liver. It refers to all forms of liver disease characterised by a significant loss of cells. This disease is quite common in old age. In France, over 20 per cent patients with cirrhosis of liver have been found to be over the age of 70 years. In the United States, in a survey it was found that the disease was at its peak in the seventh decade of life.

In cirrhosis of the liver, although regenerative activity continues, the progressive loss of liver cells exceeds cell replacement. There is also progressive distortion of the vascular system which interferes with the portal blood flow through the liver. The progressive degeneration of liver structure and function may ultimately lead to hepatic failure and death. The most common of several forms of cirrhosis is portal cirrhosis, also known as haennoc's cirrhosis.

Symptoms

In the early stages of the disease, there may be nothing more than frequent attacks of gas and indigestion, with occasional nausea and vomiting. There may be some abdominal pain and loss of weight. In the advanced stage, the patient develops a low grade fever. He has a foul breath, jaundiced skin and distended veins in the abdomen. Reddish hair like markings, resembling small spiders, may appear on the face, neck, arms and trunk. The abdomen becomes bloated and swollen, the mind gets clouded and there may be considerable bleeding from the stomach.

The clinical course of the disease in the elderly is similar to younger patients. It has, however, been found that the elderly patients with evidence of malnutrition develop considerably more severe symptoms than their younger counterparts.

Causes

Excessive use of alcohol over a long period is the most potent cause of cirrhosis of the liver. It has been estimated that one out of 12 chronic alcoholics in the United States develops cirrhosis. The disease can progress to end-stage of hepatic failure, if the person does not abstain from alcohol. Cirrhosis appears to be related to the duration of alcohol intake and the quantity consumed daily. Recent researches indicate that the average duration of alcohol intake to produce cirrhosis is 10 years and the dose is estimated to be in excess of 16 ounces of alcohol daily.

Poor nutrition can be another causative factor in the development of cirrhosis and a chronic alcoholic usually suffers from severe malnutrition as he seldom eats. Other causes of cirrhosis are excessive intake of highly seasoned food, habitual taking of quinine for a prolonged period in tropical climate and drug treatments for syphilis, fever and other diseases. It may also result from a highly toxic condition of the system in general. In fact, anything which continually overburdens the liver cells and leads to their final breakdown can be a contributing cause of cirrhosis.

Treatment

The patient should be kept in bed. He must abstain completely from alcohol in any form. He should undergo an initial liver cleaning programme with a juice fast for five to seven days. Freshly-extracted juices from red beets, lemon, papaya and grapes may be taken during this period. This may be followed by the fruit and milk diet for two or three weeks. In this regimen, the patient should have three meals a day of fresh juicy fruits and milk. The fruits may include apple, pear, grapes, grapefruit, orange, pineapple and peach. One litre of milk may be taken on the first day. It should be increased by 250 ml daily upto two litres a day. The milk should be fresh and unboiled, but may be slightly warmed, if desired. It should be sipped very slowly.

After the fruit and milk diet, the patient may gradually embark upon a well-balanced diet of three basic food groups, namely (i) seeds, nuts and grains (ii) vegetables and (iii) fruits, with emphasis on raw organically grown foods. Adequate high quality protein is necessary in cirrhosis. The best complete proteins for liver patients are obtained from raw goat's milk, home-made raw cottage cheese, sprouted seeds and grains and raw nuts, especially almonds. Vegetables such as beets, squashes, bitter gourd, egg-plant, tomato, carrot, radish and papaya are useful in this condition. All fats and oils should be excluded from the diet for several weeks.

The patient should avoid all refined, processed and canned foods, sugar in any form, spices and condiments, strong tea and coffee, fried foods, all preparations cooked in ghee, oil or butter and all meats rich in fat. The use of salt should be restricted. The patient should also avoid all chemical additives in food and poisons in air, water and environment.

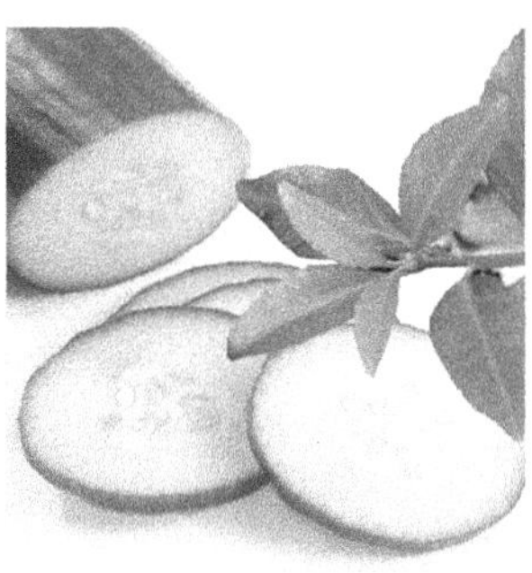

The juice of carrot, in combination with spinach juice, or cucumber and beet juice, has been found beneficial in the treatment of cirrhosis of the liver. In the first combination, 200 ml. of spinach juice should be mixed with 300 ml. of carrot juice to prepare 500 ml. or half a litre of combined juices. In the second combination, 100 ml. each of cucumber and beet juices should be mixed with 300 ml. of carrot juice.

Black seeds of papaya (papita) have been found useful in the cirrhosis of the liver, caused by alcoholism and malnutrition. A tablespoon of juice obtained by grinding the seeds, mixed with 10 drops of fresh lime juice, should be given once or twice daily for about a month as a medicine for this disease.

The herb trailing eclipta (Bhringraj), botanically known as Eclipta alba, has proved valuable in cirrhosis of the liver. The juice of all parts of this plant should be taken in doses of one teaspoon mixed with honey, three times daily.

A warm-water enema should be used during the treatment to cleanse the bowels. If constipation is habitual, all steps should be taken for its eradication. Application of alternate compress to liver area followed by general wet sheet rub will be beneficial. The morning dry firiction and breathing and other exercises should form a regular daily feature of the treatment.

CHAPTER 40

Gallbladder Disorders

The gallbladder is a pear-shaped organ, 10 cm. long and three to five cm. wide, attached to the under-surface of the liver on the right side. The main function of the gallbladder is to store the bile secreted by the liver. Bile is an excretion composed mainly of bile salts and acids, colour pigments and cholesterol. It assists in the digestion and absorption of fats and the absorption of fat-soluble vitamins A, D, E, and K, minerals and calcium.

The main problems which affict the gallbladder are an inflammatory condition known as cholecystitis and gall-stones. Gall-stones are usually caused by disturbances in the composition of the bile. A change in the ratio of cholesterol and bile salts may result in the formation of deposits. At the start, these may be in the form of fine gravels. But these fine particles constitute the nucleus for further deposits, ultimately leading to the formation of larger stones. An irritation of the lining of the gallbladder due to inflammation may also lead to the formation of particles. The incidence of gall-stones is higher in females than males, particularly in the obese.

Gallbladder disorders are common in old age. The incidence of gall-stones rises with age. About 30 per cent women and 15 per cent of men by the age of 70 in Europe and the United States develop gall-stones. In many instances, however, the elderly people do not have any symptoms and they are detected at postmortem.

Symptoms

The major symptom of gallbladder disease is acute or intermittent epigastric pain. Indigestion, gas, a feeling of fullness after meals, constipation, nausea and disturbed vision are the other usual symptoms. Intolerance to fats, dizziness, jaundice, anaemia, acne and other lesions may also occur. Varicose veins, haemorrhoids and breakdown of capillaries are also disorders associated with gallbladder troubles.

Most elderly patients with gallbladder disorders do not have any symptoms. However, when symptoms occur, they are almost similar to those found in younger age-groups. These include dyspepsia, with fatty intolerance, attacks of cholecystitis or episodes of obstructive jaundice, when stones enter the common bile duct.

Causes

The association of gallbladder disease with obesity together with their reported rarity in primitive people, living on simple diets, suggest that dietary factors play a major role in the development of this disease.

The main cause of gallbladder disorders is overnutrition caused by refined carbohydrates, especially sugar as the loss of fibre removes a natural barrier to energy intake. Overnutrition also leads to increased cholesterol secretion. Meals rich in fats may cause an attack of gallbladder pain or gall-stone colic. Chronic constipation is a most important predisposing factor. Poor health, hereditary factors, stress, spinal displacements, bad posture and muscular tension may also cause gallbladder disorders. The Chinese link the gallbladder disorders with the emotion of anger.

Types of gall-stones

There are three types of gall-stones, depending on the cause of their formation. These are: cholesterol stones, caused by the change in the ratio of cholesterol to bile salts; pigment stones, composed of bile pigment and caused by the destruction of red blood cells due to certain blood diseases, and mixed stones consisting of layers of cholesterol, calcium and bile pigment resulting from stagnation of the bile flow. The third type is by far the most common.

Treatment

Surgery becomes necessary if the gall-stones are very large or in cases in which they have been present for long. Smaller gall-stones can, however, be cleared through dietetic cure. In cases of acute gallbladder inflammation, the patient should fast for two or three days, until the acute condition is cleared. Nothing but water should be taken during the fast. After the fast, the patient should take fruit and vegetable juices for few days. Carrot, beet, grapefruit, pear, lemon or grapes may be used for juicing.

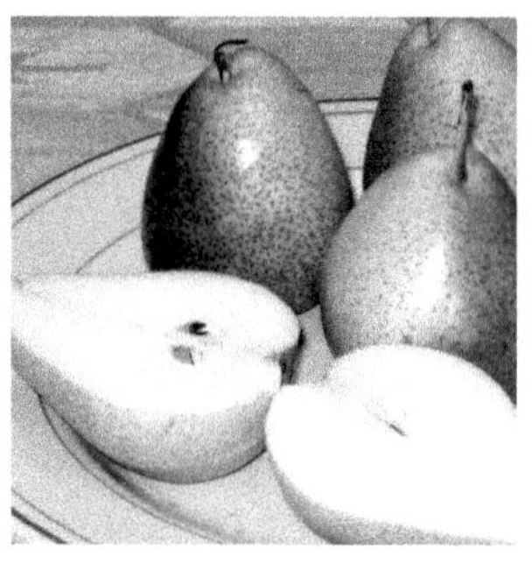

After the juices, the patient should adopt a well-balanced diet which should contain an adequate amount of all the essential nutrients. Ideally, the diet should be lacto-vegetarian, with emphasis on raw and cooked vegetables, fresh fruits and vegetable juices, and a moderate amount of fruits and seeds. Pears should be eaten generously as they have a specific healing effect on gallbladder. Yoghurt, cottage cheese and a tablespoon of olive oil twice a day should also be included in the diet. Oil serves as a stimulant for the production of bile and lipase, the fat digesting enzymes. High quality vegetable oil in the diet also prevents gall-stone formation.

The patient should avoid all meats, eggs, animal fats and processed and denatured foods as well as fried foods. The diet should also exclude refined carbohydrates, especially sugar, sugar products, alcohol, soft drinks, cakes, puddings, ice-cream, coffee and citrus fruits. The patients should eat frequent small meals rather than three large meals.

The fresh juice of beets (Chukandar), in combination with the juices of carrot and cucumber, is one of the finest cleansing material for gallbladder. This juice has proved beneficial in the treatment of all disorders relating to this organ.

The use of pear (Naspati) is another excellent remedy for gallbladder disorders. The fruit or its juice should be taken liberally by the patient with beneficial results. It exercises a special healing effect in these conditions, including gall-stones.

The flowers, seeds and roots of chicory (Kasni) or endive plant are considered valuable in gallbladder disorders. About 30 to 60 ml. of decoction of the flowers, seeds or roots can be used three times daily, with beneficial results, in the treatment of these disorders. Endive or chicory juice in almost any combination promotes the secretion of bile and is, therefore, very good for both liver and gallbladder dysfunctions.

Oil cure has been advocated by some nature cure practitioners for the removal of gall-stones. Raw, natural, unrefined vegetable oils of olive or sunflower are used. The procedure is to take one ounce of vegetable oil, preferably olive oil, first thing in the morning and follow it immediately with four ounces of grapefruit juice or lemon juice. This treatment should be taken each morning for several days, even weeks, if necessary.

The pain of gall-stone colic can be relieved by the application of hot packs or fomentation to the upper abdominal area. A warm water enema at body temperature will help eliminate faecal accumulations if the patient is constipated. Exercise is also essential.

CHAPTER 41

Jaundice

Jaundice is the most common of all liver disorders. It is a condition in which yellow discoloration of the skin and mucous membranes occurs due to an increase in the bile pigments, bilirubin, in the blood.

The bile, produced by the liver, is a vital digestive fluid which is essential for proper nutrition. It exercises a most favourable influence on the general processes of digestion. It also prevents decaying changes in food. If the bile is prevented from entering the intestines, there is an increase in gases and other products. Normally, the production of bile and its flow is constant.

There are three forms of jaundice. These are; hemolytic jaundice due to excessive destruction of red blood cells, resulting in increased bilirubin formation and anaemia; obstructive jaundice which occurs when there is a block to the pathway between the site of conjugation of bilirubin in the liver cells and the entry of bile into the duodenum; and hepatocellular jaundice, resulting from damage to liver cells either by viral infection or by toxic drugs. All the three forms are marked by yellow discoloration of the skin and the whites of the eyes. Jaundice in old age is most commonly obstructive. It is perhaps the most common single problem associated with hepatobiliary diseases in the elderly.

Symptoms

The symptoms of jaundice are extreme weakness, headache, fever, loss of appetite, undue fatigue, severe constipation, nausea and yellow coloration of the eyes, tongue, skin and urine. The patients may also feel a dull pain in the liver region. Obstructive jaundice may be associated with intense itching.

Causes

Jaundice is indicative of the malfunctioning of the liver. It may be caused by an obstruction of the bile ducts which discharge bile salts and pigment into the intestine. The bile then gets mixed with blood and this gives a yellow pigmentation to the skin. The obstruction of the bile ducts could be due to gall-stones or inflammation of the liver, known as hepatitis, caused by a virus. In the latter case, the virus spreads and may lead to epidemics owing to overcrowding, dirty surroundings, insanitary conditions and contamination of food and water. Other causes of jaundice are pernicious anaemia and certain diseases affecting the liver such as typhoid, malaria, yellow fever and tuberculosis.

Gall-stones are most often responsible for this disease in old age. It has been noted in the previous chapter how frequently gall-stones are present in the elderly and most of them do not present any symptoms. Stones may pass into the common duct and become impacted so as to cause jaundice. Mild jaundice may occur in the elderly during an attack of acute cholecystitis. It may also occur in pernicious anaemia.

Treatment

The simple form of jaundice can be cured rapidly by diet therapy and exercise. Recovery will, however, be slow in serious cases which have been caused by obstruction or pressure in the bile ducts. The patient should rest until the acute symptoms of the disease subside.

The patient should be put on a juice fast for about five days. The juices of orange, lemon, grapes, pear, carrot, beet and sugarcane can be taken. A hot water enema should be taken daily during this period to ensure regular bowel elimination, thereby preventing the absorption of decomposed, poisonous material into the blood stream. The juice fast may be continued till the acute symptoms subside.

After the juice fast, the patient may adopt an all-fruit diet for further three to five days. In this regimen, he should have three meals a day of fresh juicy fruits such as apples, pears, grapes, oranges and pineapple. Thereafter a simple diet may be resumed on the following lines:

Upon arising: A glass of warm water with juice of half a lemon.

Breakfast: One fresh juicy fruit such as apple, pear, papaya, grapes, berries and mango, one cup wheat dalia or one slice of whole meal bread.

Mid-morning: Orange or pear juice.

Lunch: Raw vegetable salad, two small chapattis of whole wheat flour, a steamed leafy vegetable such as spinach, methi saag or carrot and a glass of buttermilk.

Mid-afternoon: Coconut water or apple juice.

Dinner: One cup strained vegetable soup, two chapattis of whole meals, baked potato and one other leafy vegetable like methi or spinach.

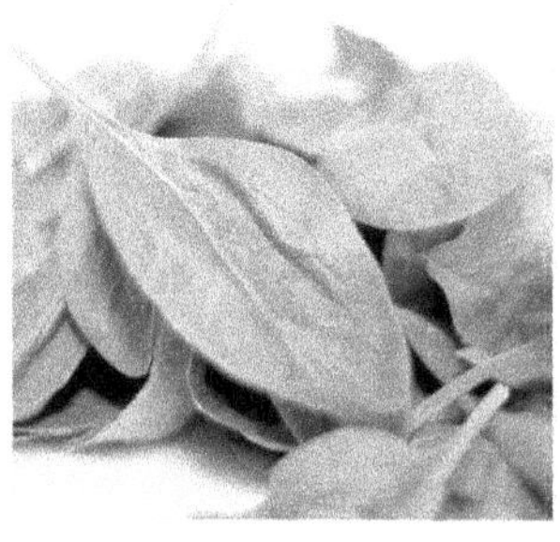

Before retiring: A glass of hot skimmed milk, with honey if desired.

All fats like ghee, butter, cream and oils must be avoided for atleast two weeks, and after that butter and olive oil may be kept down to the minimum. A light carbohydrate diet, with exclusion of fats, best obtained from vegetables and fruits should be taken.

The patient should take plenty of fresh vegetables and fruit juices. Dandelion leaves, radishes with leaves, endive should be added to daily raw vegetable salad. Raw apple and pears are especially beneficial. Barley water, drunk several times during the day, is considered a good food remedy for jaundice. One cup of barley should be boiled in three litres of water and simmered for three hours.

Digestive disturbances must be avoided. No food with a tendency to ferment or putrefy in the lower intestines like pulses and legumes should be included in the diet. Drinking a lot of water with lemon juice will protect the damaged liver cells.

The juice of bitter luffa (Karvi Torai) is regarded an effective remedy for jaundice. It is obtained by pounding and squeezing through cloth. The juice should be placed on the palm of the hand and drawn up through the nostrils. This will cause a profuse outflow of the yellow fluid through the nostrils. The toxic matter having been evacuated in a considerable quantity, the patient will feel relieved. It is, however, a strong medicine and may cause, in the patients with delicate nature, side-effects like giddiness, migraine and at times high fever for a short duration. Its use should, therefore, be avoided by such patients. If the juice of green bitter luffa is not available, it can be substituted by two to three drops of the fluid obtained by soaking its crusts overnight in water. This will produce an identical effect.

Another valuable remedy for jaundice is the green leaves of radish (Muli). The leaves should be pounded and their juices extracted through cloth. Half a litre of this juice should be taken daily by an adult patient. It should be strained through a clean piece of muslin cloth before use. It induces healthy appetite and proper evacuation of bowels and this results in gradual decrease of the trouble. In most cases, complete cure can be ensured within eight or ten days.

Tomatoes (Tamatar) are valuable in jaundice. A glass of fresh tomato juice, mixed with a pinch of salt and pepper, taken early in the morning, is considered an effective remedy for this disease.

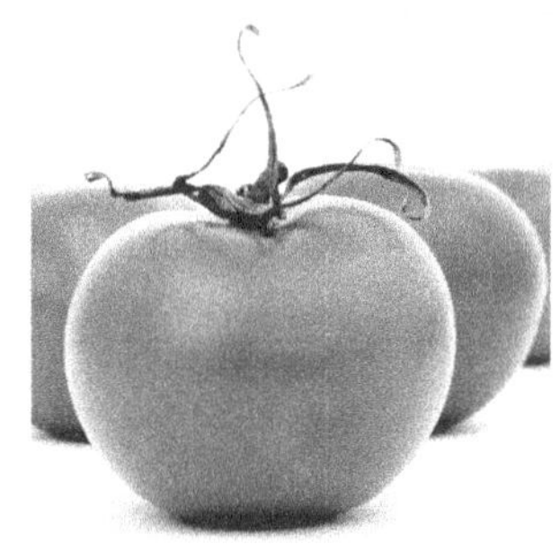

The leaves of snake gourd (Chachinda) have also been found useful in jaundice. An infusion of the leaves should be given in doses of 30 to 60 ml. mixed with decoction of the coriander seeds thrice daily in the treatment of this disease.

The jaundice patient can overcome the condition quite easily with the above regime and build up his sick liver until it again functions normally. A recurrence of liver trouble can be prevented with reasonable care in the diet and life style, with regular, moderate exercise and frequent exposure to sunshine, fresh air and adequate rest.

Research has shown that the liver has an excellent capacity to regenerate itself provided all essential nutrients are adequately supplied. Diets high in complete proteins, Vitamin C, the B Vitamins, particularly choline, and Vitamin E can hasten its regeneration. Even after recovery, it is essential to keep the diet highly adequate for a long period to prevent recurrence of the trouble.

SECTION VII

MUSCULO-SKELETON SYSTEM DISORDERS

CHAPTER 42

Osteoporosis

Osteoporosis, commonly known as soft or brittle bones, refers to increased porousness of bones. The word literally means porous or honeycombed bones. In this disorder, the bones of the skeleton become fragile due to excessive loss of tissues. It causes the bones to fracture more easily than they should. If the disease affects the spine, it may lead to the collapse of the vertebral bodies and consequent deformity.

Normal bone consists of a series of thin, intersecting plates, called 'trabeculae'. These plates are surrounded by a dense shell. These plates form, what is called the bone mass. In osteoporosis, they become filled with holes or may even totally disappear. This causes a diminution of bone mass. With loss of bone mass, the shell also becomes thin. All these changes make the bones extremely fragile and it can crack with the most trivial injury.

Ageing is invariably accompanied with loss of bone in human beings. It is associated with a progressive decline in bone strength and increase in fracture rates. Osteoporosis is thus quite common in old age, although it may occur at any age. Bone mass increases rapidly upto adolescence and continues to increase at a reduced rate until the early 30s. In women, at the menopause, there is a particularly rapid loss of bone for several years followed by a slower decline throughout the rest of life. This is attributable to estrogen deficiency that occurs after menopause. In men, bone mass declines steadily from the age of 45 onwards. There is wide individual variation. The bones commonly affected are wrist bones, ankle bones, spine and hip bones.

Symptoms

Osteoporosis is usually accompanied by severe pain. In elderly patients, the disease is accompanied by an actual loss of height and by bending causing a humpback, the deformity that crowds lungs and digestive organs. Other symptoms of osteoporosis are backache and spasms of the back muscles, aching of the long bones and thighs, thinning of the pelvic bones, loss in twisting and bending strength and frequent occurrence of spontaneous firactures.

Causes

Abnormal porosity of bones in older people results from nutritional deficiencies and the body's inability to absorb and utilise nutrients. Prolonged deficiency of calcium and Vitamin D in particular leads the skeleton to become demineralized and shrunken. Because of calcium losses during pregnancies and menstruation, the disease is far more prevalent in women than in men. A broken hip bone is usually considered to be the result of a fall. But in reality the collapse of the bone is the cause of a fall, which first draws attention to osteoporosis.

Other causes of this disease are overconsumption of meat, heavy smoking, chronic alcoholism, post-menopausal hormonal imbalances and diminished physical activity with age. Prolonged cortisone treatment, by blocking the bone-building activity and decreasing the intestinal absorption of calcium, may also cause osteoporosis.

Osteoporosis is the most common metabolic bone disease and a major health hazard in old age. It is responsible for thousands of fractures every year. In the elderly, hip fracture is the commonest cause of long term illness and death due to complications of long periods of rest in bed.

Treatment

Diet plays an important role in the treatment of osteoporosis. To begin with, the patient should adopt a raw-juice diet for about five days. In this regimen, he should take juices of fresh fruits and vegetables, diluted with water on 50:50 basis, every two hours during the day. Fruits and vegetables which can be used for juices are orange, lemon, pineapple, papaya, green leafy vegetables, red beet and carrot. A warm-water enema should be taken daily during this period to cleanse the bowels.

After the raw juice diet, the patient may gradually embark upon a well-balanced diet consisting of seeds, nuts, and grains, vegetables and fruits. The emphasis should be on mineral-rich foods such as whole grains, seeds, nuts, cooked and raw vegetables and fruits, milk and milk products such as homemade cottage cheese.

Foods rich in calcium, magnesium, potassium and silicon will be specially beneficial in the treatment of this disorder. These foods are green vegetables, cabbage, carrots, fruits and berries of all kinds, strawberries, raspberries, blueberries. Sesame seeds and sunflower seeds are excellent foods for use in this disease.

The patient should also take liberal quantities of foods rich in lactic acid, sour milk products, oats, barely, millet and rice.

The diet should be supplemented with a good all inclusive mineral and trace mineral supplement and Betaine Hydrochloride tablets with each meal to ensure proper assimilation.

The patient should avoid large meals and overeating. He should eat slowly and chew his food extremely well. He should avoid tea, coffee, fresh foods, white sugar and white flour products, processed, refined and denatured foods. Smoking and alcoholic beverages are to be completely forbidden.

Latest studies indicate that trace mineral boron can exercise great influence on osteoporosis. This mineral is found in fruits and nuts. A deficiency of boron can hamper calcium metabolism, and thereby make the bones brittle. New research shows that boron dramatically boosts blood levels of the hormone estrogen and other compounds that prevent calcium loss and bone demineralization. Boron can thus serve as a mild estrogen replacement therapy.

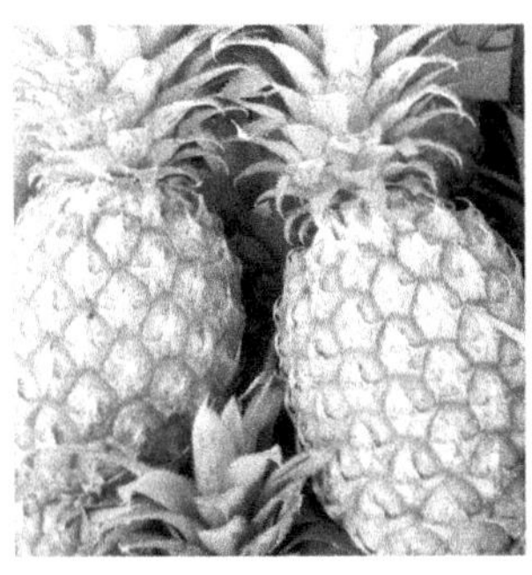

The use of pineapple is considered an effective remedy for keeping the bones strong. Dr. Jeanne Freeland-Graves, Professor of nutrition at the University of Texas at Austin, advises regular drinking of pineapple juice or eating other foods high in the trace mineral manganese to keep the bones strong. Manganese, like boron, is involved in bone metabolism. In a study, Dr. Freeland-Graves discovered that women with osteoporosis had about one-third less manganese in their blood than healthy women. Further, when given manganese, the diseased women absorbed twice as much, showing that their bodies needed it.

The patient should undertake regular physical exercise both for prevention and treatment of osteoporosis. Exercises which put stress on long bones such as walking, jogging and bicycling will be very beneficial.

CHAPTER 43

Arthritis

The word 'arthritis' means 'inflammation of joints.' It comes from two Greek words, athron meaning joints and itis meaning inflammation. It is a chronic disease process. In the early stages, the whole body is usually involved and one or two joints may becomes completely deformed, leaving the patient handicapped and somewhat weakened.

There are two categories of joints, namely, synarthrosis or those which do not move very much and do not have a cavity, and diarthrosis or those which move freely and have a joint cavity. The first type of joints are found in the head and spinal column. The second type, which is most frequently affected by arthritis, is more common and is found in the shoulders, elbows, wrists, fingers, knees, ankles and toes.

Arthritis assumed various forms, the most frequent being osteoarthritis and rheumatoid arthritis. The former is a degenerative joint disease which results from structural changes in the articular in the joints, usually those which are weight-bearing such as the spine and knees. The latter is a serious disease which affects not only the joints of the fingers, wrists, hips, knees and feet but also the muscles, tendons and other tissues of the body.

Rheumatologists believe that arthritis occurs from childhood onwards. Older people, however, have more and suffer more from it. Arthritis in old age occurs when there are already several ageing or degenerative features and it often occurs in conjunction with other diseases.

Osteoarthritis is perhaps the most important and frequent joint disease affecting the elderly. It may account for up to 90 per cent of diagnoses. Though the peak decade of onset of rheumatoid arthritis is the fifth, it is not unusual that the disease may occur for the first time in sixties or seventies. This disease is thus common in the elderly and presents with a wide spectrum of disease severity and clinical manifestations. The ravages on the joints accumulate with time, as do the effects on extra articular tissues.

Symptoms

The chief symptoms of osteoarthritis are pain and stiffness in the joints. The pain usually increases after exercise. Other symptoms include watery eyes, dry neck, leg cramps, allergies, arteriosclerosis, impairment of the functioning of the gallbladder and liver disturbances. Rheumatoid arthritis is often called the "Cooked food disease." It usually develops gradually over several months with persistent pain and stiffness in one or more joints. Ultimately the whole body is affected. Symptoms include anaemia, colitis, constipation, gallbladder disturbances, low blood pressure, deformed hands and feet.

Causes

Osteoarthritis results from structural changes in the articular cartilage in the joints, usually those which are weight bearing such as the spine and knees. Rheumatoid arthritis is due to an inflammatory process of the synovium or lining of the joints accompanied by swelling and eventual deformity. The condition may be caused by hormonal imbalance, physical and emotional stress, infection, severe fright, shock and injury. Hereditary factors may also be responsible for the onset of this disease.

Treatment

According to the modern medical system, there is no cure for arthritis and the patient must learn to live with it. Naturopathy, however, believes in dietetic cure of the disease. Most chronic arthritis patients are heavy eaters and often take food furnishing 3,500 to 4,000 calories. As they cannot utilise all the starchy elements of this intake, toxins accumulate and an excessive acid waste results in the aggravation of prevalent joint condition. A low-calorie diet, consisting of about 2,000 calories with a minimum carbohydrate content, is advisable. The diet should, however, include an adequate amount of vitamins, calcium, phosphorus and iron.

The diet of the arthritis patient should be planned along alkaline lines and should include fruits and vegetables for protection and proteins and carbohydrates for energy. It may consist of a couple of fresh raw vegetables in the form of salad and at least two cooked vegetable. Cabbage, carrot, celery, cucumber, endive, lettuce, onion, radishes, tomato, and water cress may be used for raw salad. The cooked vegetables may include asparagus, beets, cauliflower, cabbage, carrots, celery, brinjal, mushroom, onions, peas, spinach, squash, tomatoes and turnips.

In severe cases, it will be advisable to put the patient on vegetable juice therapy for about a week. Green juice, extracted from any green leafy vegetable mixed with carrot, celery and red beet juices, is specific for arthritis. The alkaline action of raw juices dissolves the accumulation of deposits around the joints and in other tissue. Fresh pineapple is also valuable as the enzyme in fresh pineapple juice, bromelain reduces swelling and inflammation in osteoarthritis and rheumatoid arthritis. Repeated juice fasts are recommended at intervals of every two months.

Certain foods are harmful for arthritis patients and these should be excluded from the diet. These include aerated waters of any kind, all cheese except cottage cheese, bacon, ham, sausages and preserved meats, pastries, cakes, pies, sweet buns and white bread, all salad dressings, all soups from meat stock, rice and white flour products. Candy, sweetmeats, sugar, ice-cream, condiments, tea and coffee should also be avoided. Fruits permitted in arthritis are apples, lemons, oranges, banana, pears, the various berries, apricot, pineapple, plums and melons.

The raw potato juice therapy is considered one of the most successful biological treatment for rheumatic and arthritis conditions. It has been used in folk medicine for centuries. The old method of preparing potato juice was to cut the potato into thin slices, without peeling the skin, and place overnight in a large glass filled with cold water. The water should be drunk in the morning on an empty stomach. Fresh juice can also be extracted from potatoes and drunk, diluted with water on 50:50 basis first thing in the morning.

Studies have shown that calcium can help in arthritis. Several patients have discovered that the joint pains have either been relieved or entirely abolished after taking calcium. This mineral should be taken in liberal quantities for at least four months to achieve beneficial results. Drinking water kept overnight in a copper container has also been found beneficial in the treatment of arthritis.

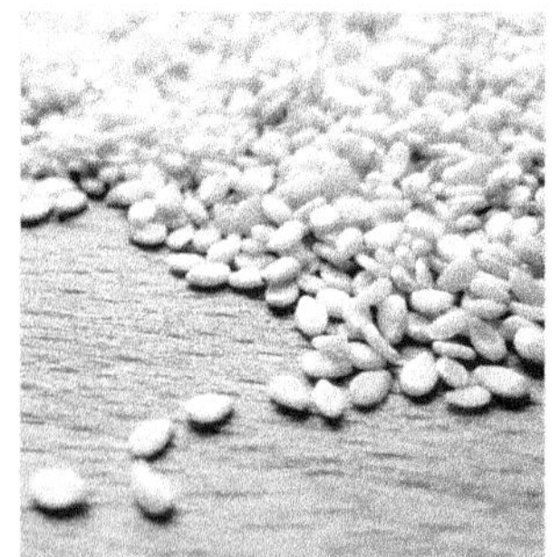

Black sesame (Til) or gingely seeds, soaked overnight in water, have been found to be effective in preventing frequent joint pains. The water in which the seeds are soaked should also be taken along with the seeds first thing in the morning.

Garlic (lahasoon) is another effective remedy for arthritis. It has shown to exhibit an anti-inflammatory property which could account for its effectiveness in the treatment of this disease.

The tea made from the herb alfalfa, especially that from its seeds has shown beneficial results in the treatment of arthritis. The patients benefit greatly by the alkalizing of food residues aided by this tea. Six or seven cups of this tea should be taken daily by arthritics for atleast two weeks.

Vitamin A and D play an important role in warding off infections, thereby preventing arthritis. Orange, papaya, carrot, whole milk and butter, all green leafy vegetables, tomatoes and raw bananas are rich in Vitamin A. Vitamin D is chiefly obtained from exposing the skin to natural sunshine. Sunlight is an important factor in the prevention of arthritis.

Constipation should be avoided as it poisons the system and adds to the irritations and inflammation of the joints. Light exercises such as walking, cycling and swimming are beneficial. Maintaining a normal body weight is also an important factor in preventing arthritis. Obesity places stress on weight bearing joints and interferes with the smooth functioning of tendons, ligaments and muscles.

The ideal yogic asanas are trikonasana, bhujangasana, shalabhasana, vakrasana and shavasana. Arthritis patients should practice these asanas regularly. Yogic kriyas like jalneti and kapalbhati and pranayamas such as anulomaviloma, ujjayi and brahmari are also beneficial.

The body should be kept warm at all times. Joints should not be bandaged tightly as this limits movement and interferes with the free circulation of blood. There should be plenty of indirect ventilation in the bedroom. Rest is of greatest importance to arthritics, who should not overdo their work, exercise or recreational activities.

CHAPTER 44

Gout

Gout refers to a form of inflammation of the joints and swellings of a recurrent type. It is associated with the presence of intracellular monosodium urate crystals in the joints. Although chronic in character, it breaks in acute attacks. Another form of gout known as pseudogout results from a deposition of crystals of calcium pyrophosphate and not urates as in true gout.

Gout was known to the physicians of ancient Greece and Rome. The classical description was written in 1663 by Sydenham, himself a life-long sufferer, who clearly differentiated it from other joint disorders. It was recognised in the 18th century that large enjoyable meals and the consumption of alcoholic drinks were often the prelude to an attack of gout.

The peak incidence of acute gout in males is usually in the fourth or fifth decade of life and it is rarely seen in women before the menopause. Over 10 per cent of patients with gout, however, experience their first attack after they have reached the age of 60 years. Pseudogout, which gives similar clinical picture to gout, occurs more commonly in the elderly. It affects large joints, in particular the knee.

Symptoms

An attack of gout is usually accompanied by acute pain in the big toe, which becomes tender, hot and swollen in a few hours. Usually, it is almost impossible to put any weight on the affected foot in the acute stage. It may also similarly affect other joints such as the knees and wrists, and sometimes more than one joint may be affected at a time. The attack usually occurs at midnight or in the early hours of the morning, when the patient is suddenly awakened. The acute attack generally lasts for a week or so. During this period the patient may run a slight fever, and feel disinclined to eat. His general health remains unaffected.

The attack may occur again after several weeks or months. The interval becomes shorter if the disease is not treated properly. The joint gradually becomes damaged by arthritis. This is chronic gout, in which chalky lumps of uric acid crystals remain in the joint and also form under the skin.

Another serious complication of gout is kidney stones containing uric acid, causing severe colic pains in the stomach. In some cases, the kidneys become damaged and do not function properly. This is a serious condition as the poisonous waste products which are normally removed by the kidneys accumulate in the blood.

Causes

The chief cause of gout is the formation of uric acid crystals in the joints, skin and kidneys. Uric acid is an end product of the body's chemical processes. Those affected by gout have a higher level of uric acid than the normal, due either to formation of increased amounts or reduced amounts of acid being passed out by kidneys in the urine. This uric acid usually remains dissolved in the blood. But when the blood becomes too full of it, the uric acid forms needle-shaped crystals in the joints which bring about attacks of gout. In case of pseudogout there is formation of crystals of calcium pyrophosphate in the joints.

Heredity is an important factor in causing this disease and

certain races are prone to gout. Other causes are excessive intake of alcoholic drinks and foods rich in protein and carbohydrate as well as lack of proper exercise. Stress is also regarded as an important cause of gout. During the alarm reaction, millions of body cells are destroyed and large quantities of uric acid freed from these cells enter the tissues after being neutralised by sodium.

The development of gout in the elderly is often secondary to an underlying disease where there is increased cellular turnover. It may also be associated with intake of certain drugs, the most common being the thiazide diuretics used for the treatment of hypertension and heart failure.

Treatment

For an acute attack, there is no better remedy than a fast. The patient should undertake a fast five to seven days on orange juice and water. Sometimes the condition may worsen in the early stages of fasting when uric acid, dissolved by juices, is thrown into the blood stream for elimination. This usually clears up if fasting is continued. In severe cases, it is advisable to undertake a series of short fasts for three days or so rather than one long fast. A warm water enema should be used daily during the period of fasting to cleanse the bowels.

After the acute symptoms have subsided, the patient may adopt an all-fruit diet for further three or four days. In this regimen, he should have three meals a day of juicy fruits such as grapes, apples, pears, peaches, oranges and pineapple. Thereafter, the patient may gradually embark upon a well balanced diet consisting of seeds, nuts and grains, vegetables and fruits, with emphasis on fresh fruits and raw vegetables.

The patient should avoid all purine and uric acid producing foods and all meats, eggs and fish. Glandular meats are especially harmful. He should also avoid all intoxicating liquors, tea, coffee, sugar, white flour and their products, all canned and processed foods. Spices and salts should be used as little as possible.

The cherry, sweet or sour, is considered an effective remedy for gout. This was discovered by Ludwig Blan some 45 years ago. Himself a gout sufferer, Blan found the use of cherries to be miraculously effective in his own case and published his own experience in a medical journal. Subsequently, many people with gout used this simple therapy with great success. To start with, the patient should consume about 15 to 25 cherries a day. Thereafter, about 10 cherries a day will keep the ailment under control. While fresh cherries are best, canned cherries can also be used with success.

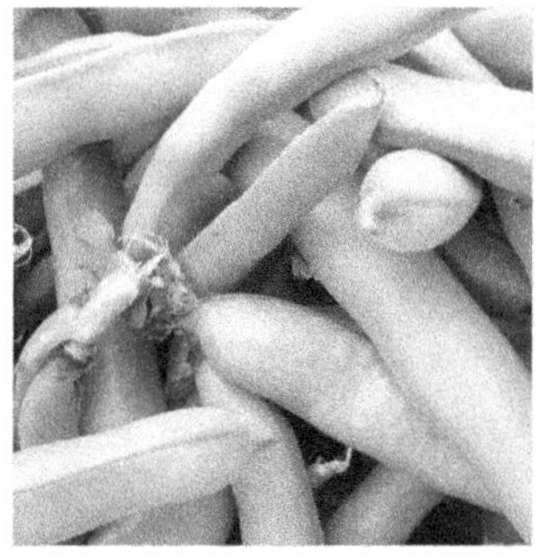

Foods high in potassium such as potatoes, bananas, leafy green vegetables, beans and raw vegetable juices are protective against gout. Carrot juice, in combination with juice of beet and cucumber juices should be mixed in 300 ml. of carrot juice to make 500 ml. of combined juice.

The juice of French or string beans has also proved effective in the treatment of gout. About 150 ml. of this juice should be taken by the patient suffering from this disease. Raw potato juice and fresh pineapple juices are also beneficial.

If the patient is overweight, he should bring his weight down by a general dietary regimen, as explained in Chapter 9 on obesity. Because of the increased risk of stones in the urinary tract, patients should maintain a good intake of non alcoholic fluids. They should drink at least eight glasses of cold or hot water daily.

The feet should be bathed in epsom salt foot baths twice daily. A quarter to half a kg. of salt may be added to a foot bath. Full epsom-salt baths should also be taken three times a week. The baths may be reduced to two per week later. Cold packs at night applied to the affected joints will be beneficial. Fresh air and outdoor exercise are also essential. The patient should eliminate as much stress from his life as possible.

CHAPTER 45

Rheumatism

The word rheumatism is derived from the Greek word "rheuma," which means a swelling. It refers to an acute or chronic illness which is characterised by pain, stiffness and swelling in muscles, bones or joints. It is a crippling disease which causes widespread invalidism, but seldom kills.

This disease usually occurs either in middle or old age and affects both men and women equally. Quite often, it may extend to the heart, resulting in the inflammation of the valves and the lining of this vital organ. It is the most common cause in 80 per cent of the cases of valvular organic diseases of the heart.

Rheumatism, perhaps, more than any other disease, although readily diagnosed, is never the same in any two persons. There are too many variations in the development of this diseases. Broadly speaking, however, it can be roughly grouped into two classes. These are muscular rheumatism which affects the muscles and articular rheumatism which affects the joints. The muscular variety is, however, far less common than that affecting the joints. In the acute form, it is found in young people, but in the chronic form, it is generally confined to the middle and old age.

Symptoms

The onset of acute types of rheumatism is characterised by

fever and rapid pulse with intense soreness and pain. In the acute muscular type, the tissues become so sensitive that even the weight of bed clothing aggravates the pain. The liver is found to be swollen. Acute rheumatism is extremely painful but it leaves no permanent defects, if treated properly. It may settle into a chronic state under a wrong mode of treatment.

The symptoms of chronic muscular rheumatism are pain and stiffness of the affected muscles. The pain increases when an effort is made to move these muscles. In case of chronic articular rheumatism, pain and stiffness are left in one or more joints of the body, with swelling in most cases. It is not usually fatal but there is a danger of permanent deformities.

Causes

The chief causes of rheumatism is the poisoning of the blood with acid wastes, which results from imperfect elimination and lowered vitality. Meat, white bread, sugar and refined cereals, to which modern man is most addicted, leave a large residue of acid toxic wastes in the system. These acid wastes are not neutralised due to absence of sufficient quantities of alkaline mineral salts in the foods eaten. This upsets the acid-alkaline balance in the body and produces the condition described as acidosis.

When there is abundant vitality, excess acids are ejected almost before they reach any appreciable concentration in one or the other of the acute cleansing efforts such as colds and fevers. When vitality is low, the acid wastes are concentrated around the joints and bony structure, where they form the basis of rheumatism. The reason why large quantities of acid wastes piling up in the system are attracted towards body structure of storage is that lime, which is the most prominent constituent of the bony structure, is an alkaline substance. In certain cases, infection from the teeth, tonsils and gallbladder may produce rheumatism. The disease is aggravated by exposure to cold weather.

Treatment

In case of acute rheumatism, the patient should be put on a short fast of orange juice and water for three or four days. The procedure is to take the juice of an orange diluted in warm water, if desired, every two hours from 8 a.m. to 8 p.m. Nothing else, whatsoever, should be taken, otherwise the purpose of the fast will be entirely lost. While fasting, the bowels should be cleansed through a warm-water enema.

After the juice fast, the patient should be placed on a restricted diet for 14 days. In this regimen, orange or grapefruit may be taken for breakfast; lunch may consist of raw salad of any vegetables in seasons, with raisins, prunes, figs or dates; and for dinner, one or two steamed vegetables such as spinach, cabbage, carrots, turnips and cauliflower and a few nuts or some sweet fruit may be taken. No bread or potatoes or other starchy food should be taken, otherwise the effect of the diet will be lost. Thereafter, the patient may gradually commence a well balanced diet of three basic food groups, namely seeds, nuts and grains, vegetables and fruits.

In case of chronic rheumatism, the patient may be placed on an all-fruit diet for four or five days. In this regimen, he should have three meals a day of fresh, juicy fruits such as apple, grapes, peach, pear, orange, pineapple and grapefruit. He may thereafter gradually adopt a well-balanced diet of three basic food groups.

The short juice fast followed by restricted diet in case of acute rheumatism and the all-fruit diet in chronic cases may be repeated at intervals of two or three months, depending on the progress being made.

The patient should take ripe fruits and fresh vegetables in abundance. Lemons are valuable and the juice of two or three lemons may be taken each day. Lots of buttermilk should be taken. The foods which should be avoided are meat, fish, white bread, sugar, refined cereals, rich, indigestible and highly seasoned foods, tea, coffee, alcohol, sauces, pickles and condiments.

The juice of raw potato (Alu) is regarded as an excellent remedy for rheumatism. One or two teaspoons of the juice pressed out of mashed raw potato should be taken before meals. This will help eliminate an acid condition and relieve rheumatism. In some rural areas in Great Britain, it is a custom for rheumatic sufferers to carry a potato in their pockets, in the belief that the potato will absorb in itself some of the acid from the sufferer's body. The old potato is thrown away and replaced by a new one after a few days.

The skin of the potato is also an excellent remedy for rheumatism. The skin is exceptionally rich in vital mineral salts and the water in which the peelings have been boiled is one of the best medicines for the ailments caused by excess of acid in the system. The potato peelings should be thoroughly washed and boiled for few minutes. The decoction should then be strained and a glass of the same should be taken three or four times daily.

Celery (Ajmuda) is another effective remedy for rheumatism. A fluid extract of the seeds is more powerful than the raw vegetable. This also has a tonic action on the stomach and kidneys. Five to ten drops of this fluid should be taken in hot water before meals. Powdered seeds can be used as a condiment.

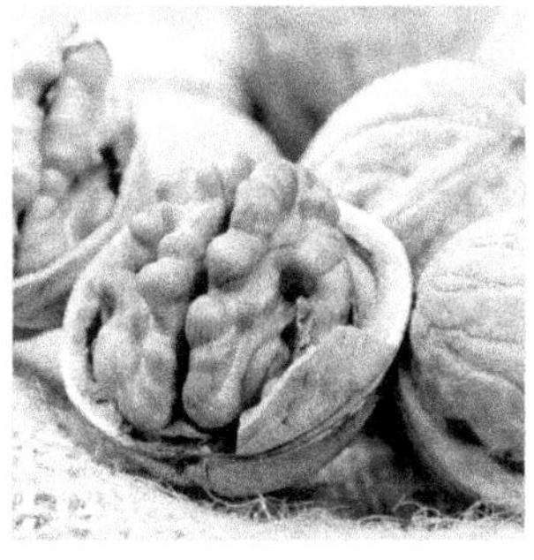

Walnuts (Akhrot) are valuable in rheumatism. They should, however, be thoroughly masticated to achieve beneficial results. About one dozen can be taken daily in the treatment of this condition. The herb rhubarb (Revand chini) has also been found valuable in rheumatism. The green stalks of this herb should be pounded with an equal quantity of lump sugar. It should be taken in quantity of a nutmeg three or four times a day. This remedy seldom fails.

Other helpful methods in the treatment of rheumatism are application of radiant heat and hot packs to the affected parts, a hot rub bath, cabinet steam bath, dry friction and sponge. The hot Epsom salt bath is also beneficial and should be taken twice a week for three months in case of chronic rheumatism and once weekly thereafter. The affected parts should also be bathed twice daily in hot water containing Epsom salt (100 gm. of salt to a bowlful of hot water) after which some olive oil should be applied. Fresh air, deep breathing and light outdoor exercises also help. Dampness and cold should be avoided.

CHAPTER 46

Muscle Cramps

Muscle cramps refer to painful spasmodic contraction of muscles in the limbs. They may occur in any of the muscles in the body. They are, however, more common in the calf of legs and feet, as in these parts of the leg, the muscles are more easily strained. It is estimated that 50 per cent of the people between the ages 15 and 80 years suffer from cramps or abnormal sensation in the legs at some stage or the other in their lives.

Leg cramps are especially prevalent in old age. They most often occur or are aggravated at night and are quite disabling. Occasionally, they are so disturbing as to cause depression in older patients.

Causes

Muscle cramps are usually caused by dietary deficiencies of vitamins and minerals, particularly of calcium, potassium, magnesium and Vitamin D and B6, or the body's inability to assimilate these nutrients from the diet. They may also result from oxygen deficiency in the tissues. Other causes of muscle cramps are mental stress, nervous irritability and other psychic factors. Muscle cramps are sometimes associated with menstrual cycle and menopausal disorders due to the influence of sex hormones on calcium metabolism.

The contributory underlying causes of muscle cramps associated with old age, where there has been adequate dietary calcium supply, are the lack of sufficient hydrochloric acid in the stomach, lack of dietary magnesium or Vitamin D, without which calcium cannot be properly utilized. Other causes include uraemia, peripheral vascular disease and neurological disability.

Treatment

Muscle cramps caused by nutritional deficiencies can be treated successfully through diet. The patient should take a diet which contains liberal quantities of all the essential nutrients. This diet may consist of seeds, nuts and whole grain, cereals, vegetables and fruits. The emphasis should be on calcium and magnesium-rich foods, such as leafy green vegetables, fresh fruits, particularly apricots, and soured milk products. The best sources of calcium are most vegetables, cereals like millet, oats, rice, sesame seeds, beans, milk and homemade cottage cheese.

The patient should avoid excess of citrus fruits, especially their juices, meats and excess of grains, especially wheat, as all of them are deficient in calcium. Millets are the best cereals for relieving muscle cramps and they should be consumed liberally by the patient. Other foods which are valuable in this disease are sesame seeds and almond, especially in the form of milk.

The use of Vitamin C and E in large doses has been found beneficial in the treatment of muscle cramps caused by oxygen deficiency in the tissue. Vitamin C has been found valuable in the assimilation of calcium in the body and preventing it from piling in the joints. Vitamin E helps circulation in the legs. Leg cramps in some cases have responded to adding vegetable oils, which is a rich source of Vitamin E, to the diet. Organic minerals, especially potassium, can be helpful in cases, where the disease is caused by mental tension and nervous disorders. Elimination of contributory psychic causes are, however, also essential in such cases.

Foot cramp may sometimes be caused by deficiency of Vitamin B6. Even many strong persons suffer from foot cramps because of lack of this Vitamin. In such cases, it is essential to take Vitamin B6 on a regular basis. This vitamin can be taken upto 50 mg daily for months together without any ill effects. It is, however, essential that while taking Vitamin B6, the whole family of Vitamin B complex should be taken simultaneously, as too much of one of the B Vitamin may cause imbalance of the other Vitamins of the B group.

Cramps associated with menstrual cycle and menopause can be treated successfully by large doses of Vitamin E, B6 and B12. Certain herbs like Indian Sarsaparilla (Magarbu or anantmue) and liquorice (mulethi) can also be used beneficially in treating such cases. Leg cramps during pregnancy can often be relieved by Vitamin B6 and calcium.

In case of cramps associated with old age due to lack of hydrochloric acid, the addition of magnesium, Vitamin D and two tablets of betaine hydrochloride after each meal can be helpful.

A useful method for relieving muscle cramps is to apply heating pad over the cramping area. Massaging the area will also be helpful. Persons suffering from leg cramps at night should keep bed covers loose, or use a foot cradle at night to keep the weight of the covers off the feet. Those sleeping on their stomach may extend their feet over the edge of the mattress to maintain a neutral foot position.

Certain exercises have been found to relieve muscle cramps. One such exercise is to lean forward, bracing against the wall with hands and arms. Keeping the heels on the floor, tilt forward to the wall until a moderate pulling sensation develops in the calf muscles. Hold the stretching position for ten seconds, stand up straight for a five second rest period of relaxation, and repeat the exercise for a total of three stretches. The exercise should be carried out three times daily.

Another exercise useful in muscle cramps is to lie fat on the back in a bed with the feet elevated for two minutes or until they become balanced. Sit on the edge of the bed with the legs dangling over for three minutes, or until the leg becomes pink. Move the feet up and down, flex the ankles in and out, massage and manipulate the toes, feet and lower legs. Lie back on the bed, cover with blankets to keep the legs warm, and rest for two minutes. This exercise should be carried out six times each, four times a day.

Low back and leg exercises assist in improving circulation to the extremities. Sit on the floor with the legs straight out in front of you, with your feet against the wall. Slowly reach for your toes with your fingers, then sit back slowly. Reach for the left foot with the right hand, then the right foot with the left hand. With hands locked behind the head, twist slowly to the right to touch the left leg with the right elbow. Return to the starting position and twist, to the left.

For relief from cramps at night, turn over in bed on your back. Point your toes toward the ceiling. This position will probably break the clutch of the cramp so that you can get back to sleep. If not, get up and walk around. If that does not help, get into a tub of hot water until the cramping subsides.

SECTION VIII

DISEASES OF THE KIDNEY AND URINARY SYSTEM

CHAPTER 47

Kidney Diseases

The kidneys are two bean-shaped organs, lying below the waist on either side of the spinal column on the back wall of the abdomen. They are soft, reddish brown in colour, and, on an average, measures 10cm, in length, 6cm, in width and is 2.5cm thick at its centre. They are the filtering plant for purifying the blood, removing water and salts from it, which are passed into the bladder as urine.

Renal function shows gradual and progressive changes with age. The kidneys become smaller in size and the nephrons become less in size and number. Basement membranes thicken and the renal arteries harden. All these changes cause fall in functional capacity of the kidney with age. The elderly have thus less reserve of renal function and are correspondingly vulnerable to the effects of disease.

One of the most serious kidney diseases is nephritis, also known as glomerulonephritis. It is most common kidney disease in the elderly as well as other age groups. It may be either acute or chronic. A synonym for nephritis is Bright's disease, for Bright (1789-1858) described examples of many different diseases which can be included under the term.

This diseases most often strikes in childhood or adolescence. It can become progressively worse and results in death, if not treated properly in the initial stage. In the alternative, it may subside into a chronic stage where the patient gets better but not often well.

Symptoms

The main symptoms of acute nephritis are pain in the kidneys, extending down to the ureters, fever, dull pain in the back and scanty and highly coloured urine. Often the urine may contain blood, albumin and casts consisting of clumps of red and white cells which come from the damaged kidneys. The patient suffers from puffiness in the face and swelling of the feet and ankles.

In the chronic stage of nephritis, which may drag on for many years, the patient passes large amounts of albumin in the urine. Later, there may be rise in blood pressure and the patient may develop uraemia. There may be frequent urination, especially during night.

Causes

Nephritis usually follows some streptococcus infection of the throat or an attack of scarlet fever or rheumatic fever. The underlying causes of nephritis are, however, the same as for diseases of the kidneys in general, namely, wrong feeding habits, excessive drinking, the suppressive medical treatment of former diseases, the habitual use of chemical agents of all kinds for the treatment of indigestion and other stomach disorders and frequent use of aspirin and other pain-killers. Nutritional deficiencies can also lead to nephritis. When Vitamin B6 and magnesium are under supplied, the kidneys are damaged by sharp crystals of oxalic acid combined with calcium. The disease also occurs if Vitamin E is deficient.

Treatment

The safest treatment for acute nephritis is fasting on raw juices. By means of the juice fast, the toxins and systemic impurities responsible for setting up of the inflammatory kidney conditions are removed rapidly. The patient should resort to juice fasting for five to seven days till the acute symptoms subside. Mostly vegetable juices such as carrot, celery and cucumber should be used during this period. A warm water enema should be taken each day while fasting to cleanse the bowels of the toxic matter being thrown off by the self-cleansing process resulting from the fast.

After the juice fast, the patient may adopt an all-fruit diet for four or five days. Juicy fruits such as apple, grapes, orange, pear, peach and pineapple should be taken during this period. Thereafter the patient may adopt fruits and milk diet for further five days. In this regimen, milk may be added to the fruit diet. After the fruit and milk diet, the patient may gradually embark upon a well-balanced low-protein vegetarian diet, with emphasis on fresh fruits and raw and cooked vegetables.

In case of chronic nephritis, a short juice fast for three days may be undertaken. Thereafter, a week or 10 days may be spent on a restricted diet. In this regimen, oranges or orange juice may be taken for breakfast. Lunch may consist of salad of two vegetable in season and dinner may comprise one or two vegetables steamed in their own juices and a few nuts. Thereafter, the patient may gradually adopt a well-balanced low-protein vegetarian diet.

Further short juice fasts, followed by a week on the restricted diet, should be undertaken at intervals of two or three months until such time as the kidney condition has shown sign of normalisation. The patient should avoid foods rich in oxalic acid such as spinach, chocolate and cocoa, Garlic, parsley, cucumber and celery are excellent vegetables. Best fruits are papaya and bananas. A small amount of soured milks and home-made cottage cheese can be included in

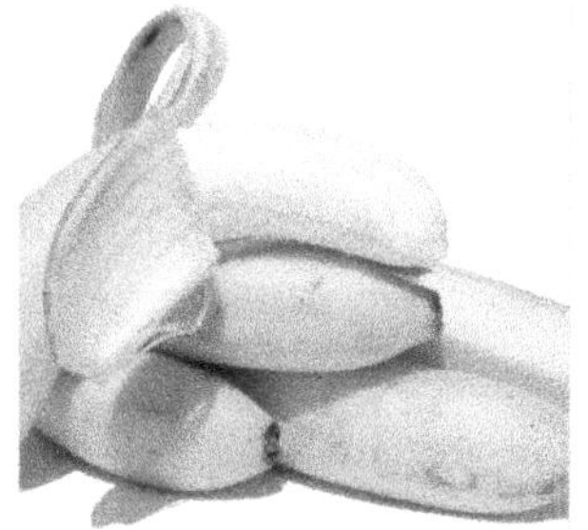

the diet. All salt should be eliminated from the diet. Five or six small meals should be taken in preference to a few large ones.

The diet should be adequate in all essential nutrients. Supplements should be given to furnish the nutrients not obtained from food. The supplements may include one tablespoon of lecithin, 30mg. of Vitamin B6, 25,000 units of Vitamin A and 300 to 600 units of Vitamin E.

Smoking and drinking, where habitual, must be completely given up. Studies have shown that smoking impairs kidney function. The patient should avoid white bread, sugar, cakes, pastries, puddings, refined cereals, greasy, heavy or fried foods. He should also avoid tea, coffee, all fresh foods, condiments, pickles and sauces.

The use of carrot juice is one of the most effective home remedies for nephritis. A glass of this juice should be taken, mixed with a tablespoon of honey and a teaspoon of fresh lime juice, every day, first thing in the morning.

The use of bananas is another effective remedy for nephritis. It is due to their low protein and salt contents and high carbohydrates content. They exercise healing effect on the kidneys. A diet of bananas only can be taken for three or four days, consuming eight to nine bananas a day in the treatment of this disease.

The use of avacado is valuable as a staple food in nephritis. The usefulness of this fruit arises from its small protein content, with none of the poisonous extractives, always present in fresh foods.

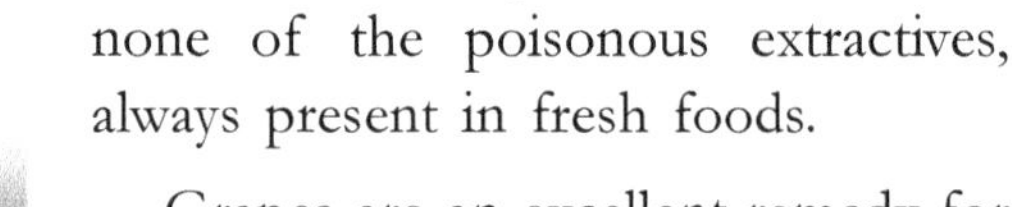

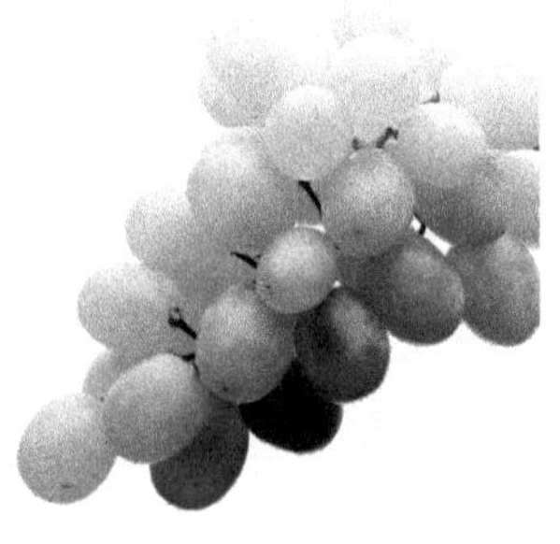

Grapes are an excellent remedy for both acute and chronic nephritis. They possess an exceptional diuretic value on account of their high contents of water and potassium, salt. Their value in kidney troubles like nephritis is enhanced by their low albumin and sodium chloride content. Tender coconut water is another valuable remedy for this disease. It can be taken beneficially once or twice a day. It acts as a very effective but safe diuretic.

All measures should be adopted to relieve the kidneys of work by increasing elimination through other channels. Hot Espom salt bath should be taken every alternate day to induce elimination through the skin as much as possible.

Fresh air and outdoor exercises will be of great benefit in all cases of nephritis and where possible, the patient should have a walk for at least three kilometers once or twice daily. The sufferer from chronic nephritis should never exert himself when doing anything. He should avoid all hurry and excitement. He should also avoid late hours.

CHAPTER 48

Bladder Infection

The bladder is one of the principal structures in the urinary system. It is situated in the lower abdomen, in the pelvis, guarded in front by bones. The body is relieved of the greater part of the waste matter, resulting from the complex working of the whole body's vital processes, by means of kidneys and bladder.

Bladder infection or cystitis is a common disease of the urinary system. Escherichia coli infections are considered the primary culprit in this disease. It is a fairly common condition in old age. The women suffer more from bladder infection as the female anatomy makes it convenient for E. coli bacteria, which normally inhabit the colon, to travel from the rectum to the vagina, up the urethra and into the bladder. This diseases is rarely dangerous but it is generally a forerunner to more serious troubles.

Certain age-related structural changes in the genito-urinary tract contribute to the high incidence of infection in the elderly. In men, enlargement of the prostate gland and associated obstruction generally causes pooling of urine in the bladder, which then becomes site for infection.

Symptoms

Bladder infection is characterised by symptoms which may cause great discomfort. The patient complains of frequency and burning on urination as well as an almost continual urge to void. There may be a feeling of pain in the pelvis and lower abdomen. The urine may become thick, dark and stringy. It may have an unpleasant smell and may contain blood or pus. The 'scalding sensation' on passing urine indicates that the inflammation has spread to the urethra. Some pain in the lower back may also be felt in certain cases. In an acute stage, there may be a rise in body temperature.

Causes

Bladder infection may result from infections in other parts adjacent to the bladder such as the kidneys, the urethra and the vagina. Local irritation and inflammation of the bladder may be caused if urine is retained there for an unduly long time. It may also result from severe constipation.

Continual draining of pus and germs from an infected kidney may injure the epithelial lining of the bladder. Trouble may also arise from the presence of the stone in either bladder or kidney. Major surgical procedures within the pelvis may lower the resistance of the bladder wall and predispose to the development of infection. Uncontrolled diabetes can also lead to this disease.

Treatment

At the onset of acute bladder infection, it is essential to withhold all solid food immediately. If there is fever, the patient should fast either on water or tender coconut water for three or four days. If there is no fever, raw vegetable juices, especially carrot juice, diluted with water on 50:50 basis, should be taken every two hours. It is advisable to rest and keep warm at this time.

Pain can be relieved by immersing the pelvis in hot water, or alternatively by applying heat to the abdomen, using a towel wrung out in hot water, covering it with dry towel to retain warmth. Care should be taken to avoid scalding. A little vegetable oil gently rubbed into the skin, will avoid too much reddening. This treatment may be continued for three or four days, by which time the inflammation should have subsided and the temperature returned to normal.

For the next two or three days, only ripe sub-acid fruits may be taken three times at five-hourly intervals daily.

These fruits may include grapes, pear, peach, apple and melon as available.

Hot and cold compresses are valuable in the treatment of bladder infection. Hot compresses relieve the pain, and cold water compresses relieve pelvic congestion and increase the activity of the skin. Care should, however, be taken to ensure that compresses do not cause chilling.

After the all-fruit diet, the patient may gradually embark upon a well-balanced diet, consisting of seeds, nuts and grains, vegetables and fruits. The patient should avoid refined carbohydrates and salt, both at table and in cooking. Salt disturbs the balance of electrolytes and tends to raise blood pressure, which is frequently already raised in kidney troubles. The diet should exclude meat, fish and poultry.

In case of chronic cystitis, the patient should commence the treatment by strict adherence to the dietary programme, designed to cleanse the blood and other tissues and at the same time provide a rich source of natural vitamins and minerals in balanced proportions. The patient may adopt the following restricted diet for seven to ten days:

Upon arising: A glass of unsweetened apple juice or carrot juice.

Breakfast: Fresh fruits, selected mainly from apple, pear, grapes, melon, peach and pineapple and a glass of buttermilk, sweetened with a little honey.

Mid-morning: Tender coconut water.

Lunch: A salad of raw vegetables such as carrot, beetroot and cabbage, mixed with curd and a teaspoon of honey. This may be followed by a ripe apple.

Mid-afternoon: One cup of unsweetened grape juice.

Dinner: A salad of green leafy vegetables and a fresh fruit, preferably a portion of melon, sweetened with a teaspoon of honey.

Before retiring: One glass of mixed raw carrot and beetroot juice.

After the restricted diet, the patient should gradually embark on a well-balanced diet consisting of seeds, nuts and grains vegetables and fruits. Even after the recovery from chronic condition, it would be advisable for the individual to live exclusively on vegetables or on tender coconut water or raw vegetable juices for a day or two, every month. The water treatment and other health building methods should, however, be continued to the greatest extent possible, so that the patient may stay cured.

The use of cucumber (Khira) juice is one of the most important home remedies found beneficial in the treatment of bladder infection. It is a very effective diuretic in this condition. A glass of this juice, mixed with two teaspoons of honey and a tablespoon of fresh lime juice, should be given three times daily.

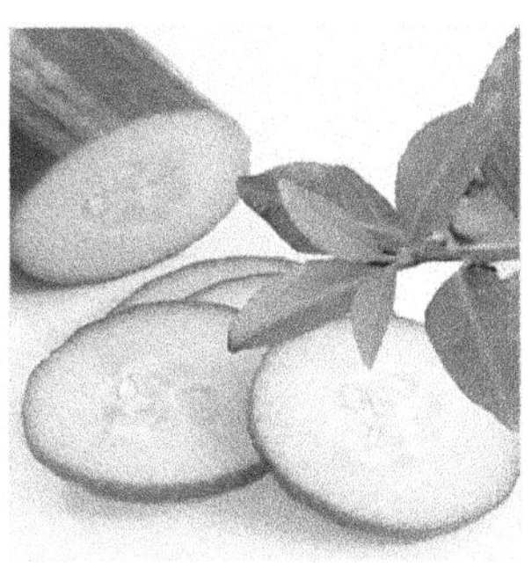

Fresh juice of the flowers of drumstick (Sanjana) is another effective remedy for bladder infection. For better results, this juice should be given twice daily with tender coconut water. It acts as a diuretic medicine in the treatment of this disease.

The juice of radish (Muli) leaves is valuable in bladder infection. A cup of this juice should be given once daily for a fortnight. Fresh lady's fingers (bhindi) is another useful vegetable in this disease. Its decoction should be taken daily.

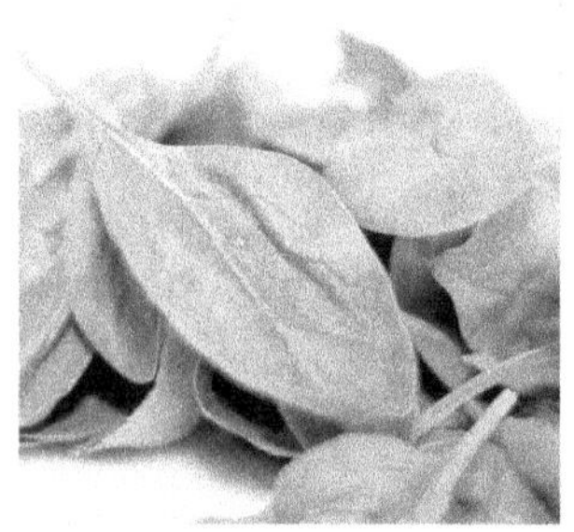

Fresh spinach (palak) juice, taken with tender coconut water on 50:50 basis once or twice a day, is considered beneficial in the treatment of bladder infection. It acts as a very effective and safe diuretic due to the combined action of both nitrates and potassium. Lime (Niboo) has also proved valuable in bladder infection. A teaspoon of lime juice should be put in 180ml. of boiling water. It should then be allowed to cool and 60 ml. of this water should be given every two hours from 8 a.m. to 12 noon in the treatment of this condition. It gives relief to burning sensation and also stops bleeding.

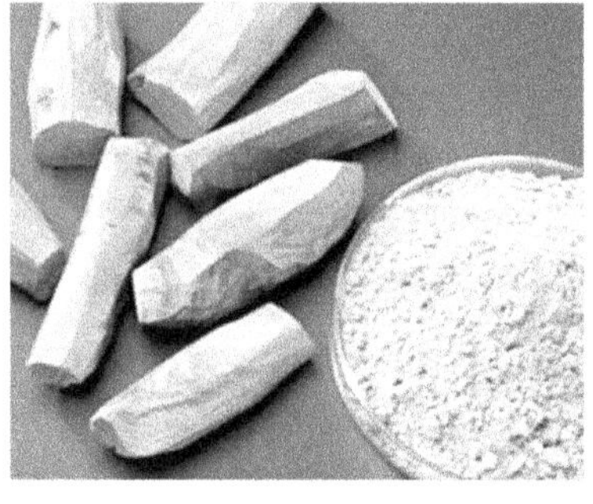

The oil of sandalwood (Chandan) is also considered valuable in this disease. This oil should be given in doses of five drops in the beginning and gradually increased to 10 to 30 drops. The efficacy of this oil can be increased by the addition of ajwain water or infusion of ginger.

CHAPTER 49

Prostate Disorders

The prostate gland is a part of the male reproductive system. It is comparable in shape and size to a large chestnut. It is reddish brown in appearance. It measures approximately one and a half inches in width and about an inch in length and weighs approximately 25 grams. It is situated at the base of the urinary bladder and around the commencement of the urethra, the membranous tube for the passage of the urine. It is thus vital in relation to emptying of the bladder and bears a close relationship to the rectum.

The prostate gland is composed of both muscular and glandular tissues. It is firmly attached to the pelvis by a dense fascial sheath. Like all muscular and glandular tissues in the body, it is adequately supplied with blood vessels, arteries, veins and nerves. The gland plays an important role in normal sexual life and its function is to secrete a fluid which is added to semen during sexual intercourse.

Nearly one-third of all men over 50 years suffer from prostate troubles of one form or another. The percentage rises with age and reaches 75 after the age of 80 years. Prostate and bladder disorders can lead to numerous other ailments such as arthritis, kidney disorders and uremia. It is, therefore of utmost importance to detect the disease in its early stages and commence treatment.

There are various types of prostate disorders. Of these, the most important are prostatitis or inflammation in the prostate gland and hypertrophy or enlargement of the prostate gland. Prostatitis may be acute or chronic. It is a painful and distressing disorder, but can be cured with proper treatment, without any adverse effects.

Enlargement of the prostate gland or hypertrophy is the most common complaint affecting the gland. This occurs mostly in men of middle or advanced age. The enlargement develops so gradually over a long period that it often assumes serious proportions before it is detected.

Symptoms

There are two warning signals to indicate the possibility of prostate disorders. The first is the interference with the passage of urine and the second is the need to void the urine frequently during the night's sleep. Other symptoms are a dull aching pain in the lower back and pain in the hips, legs and feet.

Prostate enlargement affects the glandular system as a whole. The patient experiences all the symptoms of disturbed health such as lack of energy and physical, mental and nervous disturbances.

Causes

The position of the prostate gland makes it liable to congestion and other disorders. In an erect position, pressure falls on the pelvic region just where the prostate gland is situated. With ageing, the body gets heavier and loses its flexibility which makes the pressure on the pelvis even greater and increases the vulnerability of the prostate gland. Prolonged periods of sitting down, as in certain occupations, also increases the pressure on the pelvic region resulting in congestion of the tissues in and around the prostate gland. With the passage of time, changes such as inflammation or enlargement occur in the gland.

Acute prostatitis may also result from exposure to cold and chill and from an infectious disease. Chronic prostatitis is an after-effect of the acute condition. It may also result from continual irritation of the gland due to excessive sexual excitement.

Another important cause of prostate disorders is constipation. In constipation, the faeces become hardened and the rectum or lower bowel overloaded. This causes undue pressure on the prostate gland. It also entails a great deal of straining at stool and this adversely affects the prostate gland due to its proximity to the rectum.

Treatment

The natural treatment for prostate enlargement consists of detoxicating the system by proper fasting and diet. To begin with, the patient should forgo all solid foods and subsist on orange juice and water only, for two or three days. The intake of water should be as plentiful as possible. The water may be taken cold or hot and it should be taken every hour or so when awake. This will greatly increase the flow of urine.

A warm water enema should be taken once daily during this period to clear the lower bowel of accumulations. After thorough cleansing of the bowels, hot and cold applications may be used directly on the prostate gland and its surrounding parts. The heat relieves the tissues and a brief cold immersion tones them up. The patient should also take alternate hot and cold hip baths. These are of great value in relieving pain and reducing congestion. While taking hip baths, it should be ensured that the buttocks and pelvis are well covered with water. The hot bath should be taken first for 10 minutes, followed by cold bath for one minute only.

After the short juice fast, the patient should adopt an all-fruit diet for three days. The fruits should include apple, pear, orange, grape-fruit, grapes, sweet lime, mango, melon and all other juicy fruits. This will help to clear toxins from the body and will also enable excess fat to be reduced to some extent.

The exclusive fruit diet should be followed by a restricted diet comprising two meals of fruits and one of cooked vegetables for further seven days. The vegetable meal should be taken in the evening and could consist of all kinds of cooked vegetables, preferably steam cooked. The short juice fast, followed by an all-fruit diet and a further period on fruits and vegetables may be repeated after two or three months if necessary depending on the progress being made.

Heavy starches, sweet stimulants and highly seasoned foods are entirely forbidden, as they cause direct irritation on the prostate gland and bladder. The diet should also exclude spices, condiments, salt in excess, sauces, red meats, cheese, greasy or fired foods, alcohol, tobacco and too much tea or coffee. The patient should avoid hurried meals and must chew his food thoroughly and slowly. Water should be taken between meals and not at mealtime.

Pumpkin (Kumera) seeds have been found to be an effective home remedy for prostate problems. These seeds are rich in unsaturated fatty acids which are essential to the health of the prostate.

The use of zinc has been found valuable in several cases of prostate disorders. About 30 mg. of this mineral should be taken daily in the treatment of these diseases.

Vitamin E has proved to be an important factor for prostate health. The patient should therefore use vitamin E-rich foods liberally or take 600 I.U. of this vitamin daily. Vitamin E-rich foods are whole grain products, green leafy vegetables, eggs, milk and all whole raw or sprouted seeds.

Hot and cold applications are highly beneficial in the treatment of prostate disorders. After thorough cleansing of the bowels through warm water enema, hot and cold applications may be used directly on the prostate gland and its surrounding parts. The heat relieves the tissues and a brief cold immersion tones them up. The patient should take alternate hot and cold hip baths. These are of great value in relieving pain and reducing congestion.

Wet girdle pack is another valuable remedy in the realm of hydrotherapy which provides great relief in prostatitis and prostate enlargement. For this mode of treatment, a thin cotton underwear and another thick or woolen underwear are required. The thin underwear should be wrung in cold water and worn by the patient. The thick dry underwear should be worn above the wet underwear. This treatment should be continued for 90 minutes regularly every night. If the patient feels chill, he should be covered with a blanket.

Correcting bad posture and exercise are of utmost importance in treating prostate disorders. One of the best posture-correcting methods is to lie flat on the floor at the end of the day. It gradually straightens out the back, pushes the neck into its normal position and takes the weight off the feet so that they may relax. Lie in this position for about 10 minutes till the lower part of the back begins to ache due to the strain placed on the pelvic muscles. This strain can be reduced by drawing the feet up to the buttocks. This position also takes the strain off the abdominal muscles and allows the contents of the abdomen to move more freely than in the standing position. This movement can be increased by deep breathing, and the diaphragm will then tend to pull the abdominal organs up towards the chest. Breathing in this way releases the tension on the back, lifts the pelvic organs and restores the proper angle to the ribs.

The patient should now be in a fairly relaxed state with the back resting comfortably on the floor, the neck straight and the breathing easy and full. The next position is to raise the pelvic part of the body as high as possible, and to put under it a hard cushion that will hold it as comfortably high as possible, Rhythemic breathing may be continued so as to stimulate the movements of the inner organs. The patient may also try consciously to relax and contract the abdominal muscles. This position is of great value in taking the weight and strain off the bladder and the prostate gland, and should be held for about 10 minutes or even longer, if possible. This position may be usefully varied by taking the cushion or support from under the buttocks and then raising the pelvis up and down slowly as an exercise.

Now assume the first position of lying completely flat on the back with the legs extended flat on the floor. Bend the knees, and bring them up as high as possible towards the head. Place the hands on the outside of the knees, and then pull the knees as high as they will come.

Kicking an imaginary object in this position is a very good exercise in prostate disorder. The procedure is to release the hands from the knees, and shoot out both legs, as though kicking an imaginary object suspended in the air. Do not do this too vigorously at first because it is apt to strain the abdominal muscles; but after a while a certain control will be developed over the movement, and it may be done with a good deal of speed. It is a very useful exercise, as it tends to shake up the contents of the pelvis and the jerk of the feet transmits an upward force through that region. The good effect of this movement is to activate a sluggish bowel. It should be repeated several times, according to the strength and energy of the patient.

Other moderate exercises like walking are also must. The movement of muscles and organs in the pelvis cavity during walking helps circulation to and from the gland.

The patient should avoid sexual excess, irregularities in eating and drinking, long periods of sitting and vigorous exercise. He should guard against constipation by taking plenty of fruits, bran and nuts. All efforts should be made to tone up the general condition of the body.

With a general improvement in health, the condition will be greatly relieved. Surgery should be resorted to only if the condition does not improve even after the dietary treatment and other measures outlined here.

CHAPTER 50

Sexual Impotence

Sex plays an important role in shaping human lives. It is now realised that the sex impulse is present in various forms from the earliest months until the end of life. Being a basic instinct like hunger, its satisfaction is essential for sustained harmony and well-being.

The sexual act not only quietens the excitement which is a natural occurrence during maturity, but also refreshes the body and mind. It also contributes to mental development. In fact, it exercises powerful influence upon every organ and cell and every physical and chemical process, including the nervous system.

Sexual activity, however, demands complete concentration and relaxation. It cannot be performed in haste and tension. The modern men who are usually tense and over-occupied are unable to follow these norms. Many persons, therefore, suffer from sexual dysfunctions in the male. It can be defined as failure to obtain an erection or maintain it for a reasonable length of time without attaining orgasm. The main causes of impotence are fatigue, devitalised condition of the system in general, abuse or misuse of the sexual organism over a long period, glandular deficiencies, infectious diseases including venereal diseases and psychological factors.

Impotence can be defined as the failure to have an erection in at least 25% of attempts or inability to maintain erection for penetration or an erection without sufficient rigidity for vaginal penetration. Most men experience failure occasionally. However, when they recur on a regular basis, it can have devastating effects on both the man and his partner.

The male reaches his peak of sexual activity in his teens. Thereafter a slight decline usually begins to take place.

This decline occurs so slowly over a long span of years, that its progress goes unnoticed until the fear of middle age begins. The effects of this fear are far more damaging than the results of actual ageing. In persons, who enjoy good physical and mental health, age has no effect on their sexual potency. The experts now are in unanimous agreement that continued sexual performance until late in life depends almost entirely upon health and attitude.

It may be relevant to point out that erection occurs by sexual arousal, stimulated by touch, hearing, sight, smell and from thoughts; nerve impulses that adjust hormone levels and control muscles and arteries, allowing blood to engorge the penis and make it firm; and proper blood flow.

Symptoms

Impotence takes three forms. There is primary impotence when the man's erectile dysfunction is there from the very beginning of sexual activity and he simply cannot raise an erection. This is a rare manifestation of the problem. Secondary impotence is the commonest and this implies that the man can normally attain an erection but fails on one or more occasions in between normal activity. The third form associated with age is a continuous and serious form with poor prognosis.

Causes

Since erection is the result of erotic excitement, intact nervous pathways and adequate hormonal functioning, the pathological causes of impotence are numerous. It may occur as a result of psychological illness such as depression, which lowers both sexual drive and erectile function, tiredness, alcohol abuse, the therapeutic use of estrogens, paralysis of parasympathetic nerves by drugs or permanent damage to them and diabetes. Other causes of impotence are abuse or misuse of the sexual organism over a long period and a devitalised condition of the system in general.

However, the main problem of secondary impotence is the apprehension created by failure which generates a good deal of anxiety for the next time round regarding the likelihood of failure. If, in fact, intercourse is attempted again and the same failure results, then a vicious circle is established. Anxiety of failure is established as an anticipatory reflex which in turn impairs the capacity of the penis.

Treatment

Taking of drugs or so called "remedies" in case of impotence is not only useless but dangerous. Diet is an important factor in these conditions. To begin with, the patient should adopt an exclusive fresh fruit diet from five to seven days. In this regimen, he can have three meals a day, at five hourly interval, of fresh juicy fruits such as grapes, oranges, apples, pears, peaches, pineapple and melon. The bowels should be cleansed daily during this period with a warm-water enema.

After the all-fruit diet, the patient may gradually embark upon a balanced diet of seeds, nuts and grains, vegetables and fruits with generous use of special rejuvenative foods such as whey, soured milks, particularly made from goat's milk, millet, garlic, honey, cold-pressed vegetable oils and brewer's yeast. The patient should avoid in future smoking, alcohol, tea, coffee and all processed, canned, refined and denaturated foods, especially white sugar and white flour and products made therefrom.

Certain foods are panacea for impotence. The most important

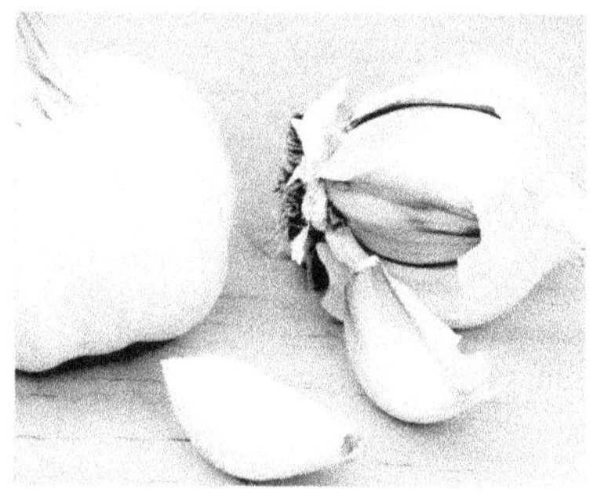

of these is the garlic (lahsoon). It is a natural and harmless aphrodisiac. According to Dr. Robinson an eminent sexologist of America, garlic has a pronounced aphrodisiac effect. It is a tonic for loss of sexual power from any cause and for sexual debility and impotency resulting from sexual over-indulgence and nervous exhaustion.

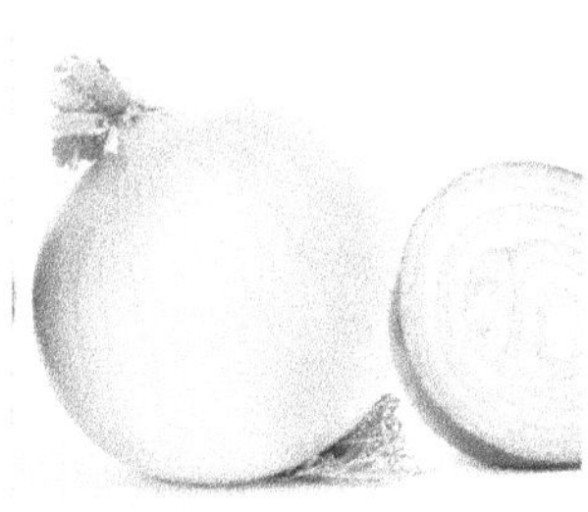

Onion (pyaz) is another most important aphrodisiac food. It stands second only to garlic. It increases libido and strengthens the reproductory organs. The white variety of onion, is, however, more useful.

Carrot (gajar) is also considered useful in impotence. For better results, carrot should be taken with half boiled egg dipped in a tablespoonful of honey once daily for a month or two. This recipe increases sex stamina by releasing sex hormones and strengthen the sexual plexus. It is for this reason that carrot halwa, prepared according to Unani specifications, is considered a very effective tonic to improve sexual strength.

The lady's finger (bhindi) is another great tonic for improving sexual vigour. It has been mentioned in the ancient Indian literature that the persons who take five to 10 grams of root powder of this vegetable with milk and 'misri' daily will never lose sexual vigour.

The dried dates is a highly strengthening food. Pounded and mixed with almonds, pistachio nuts and quince seeds, it forms an effective remedy for increasing sexual power.

Black raisins (manaqqa) are also useful for restoration of sexual vigour. They should be boiled with milk water after washing them thoroughly in tepid water. This will make them swollen and sweet. Starting with 30 grams of raisins with 200 milliliter of milk, three times daily, the quantity of raisins should be gradually increased to 50 grams each time.

Vigorous massage all over the body is highly beneficial in the treatment of impotence as it will revive the muscular vigour which is essential for nervous energy. The nerves of the genital organs are controlled by the pelvic region. Hence cold hip bath for 10 minutes in the morning or evening will be very effective.

Every effort should be made to build up the general health-level to the highest degree and fresh air and outdoor exercise are essential for the success of the treatment. Yogasanas such as dhanurasana, sarvangasana and halasana are also highly beneficial.

The scheme of treatment outlined above will go a long way in restoring sexual function, but, of course, the results achieved will depend upon the age and condition of the sufferer. Long-standing cases will obviously not get such good results from the treatment as comparatively early cases.

Where the trouble is of psychological origin, treatment should be just the same, but in these cases advice from a qualified psychotherapist would be desirable. The patient also requires a little gentle handling by a willing partner.

CHAPTER 51

Vaginitis

The elderly female may encounter a wide range of gynaecological disorders. Atrophic or 'senile' vaginitis is one of the most common problems which is particular to post menopausal women. This represents atrophy of the vaginal epithelium consequent upon the lowering of oestrogen levels after the menopause. Changes also occur in the vaginal flora so that secretions loose the acidity which protects the vagina from infection in younger women. Secondary infection is thus far more common in elderly women who may complain of pain, pruritus or of discharges which may be bloodstained.

Vaginitis can be described as an inflammation of the vagina and vulva. This can be avoided by taking proper treatment in the initial stage itself. But women usually tend to hide this problem.

The normal healthy women usually do not suffer from the sensations of itching, burning, pain or irritation. In unhealthy women and in abnormal conditions, the resident organisms (bacteria) multiply rapidly and produce excessive waste products. It causes tissue irritation in this region leading to itching, swelling and burning. There is increase in the frequency of urine which is accompanied with an unpleasant odour.

Symptoms

The symptoms of vaginitis are feeling of heat and fullness in the vagina, a dragging feeling in the groin, increased urinary frequency and vaginal discharge, that is, leucorrhoea. The clear or white secretion becomes purulent and yellow. The severity of leucorrhoea depends upon the degree of bacterial infection.

Causes

The main causes of vaginitis are irritation of vagina by external factors, like cuts, abrasions in this region, constant wearing of tight fitting clothes and wearing unclean clothes, using dirty or infected water and lack of hygiene.

Certain medications and treatments can increase susceptibility to infection. These include the use of antibiotics, hormones and excessive douching. Susceptibility is greater in cases of pregnancy, diabetes, and certain psychological condition as well as during the latter half of the menstrual cycle. Irritation from contraceptive devices can also lead to this condition.

Unhygienic conditions combined with wrong dietary habits increase toxemia thereby lowering body resistance. Whenever the body is loaded with toxins or morbid matter, it tries to eliminate it through the eliminative organs. In women, this elimination is established in the form of profuse discharge, that is leucorrhoea, initially. In later stages, the discharge can become offensive in cases of chronic inflammation.

Treatment

Maintenance of hygienic conditions is the most important factor in the treatment of vaginitis. It is only after this is achieved that morbidity and consequent inflammation and discharge can be prevented.

Another important factor is diet. The patient should fast for three to five days. Depending upon the condition, the fasting period may be extended. During this period, she may take juices of lemon and other sub-acidic fruits. This will give the system an opportunity to divert its vital energies to check inflammation and infection.

After the juice fasting, the patient may adopt a restricted diet, consisting of raw vegetable salads, fruits and sprouts. This will ensure minimal mucous secretions. This restricted diet should be continued for 10 to 15 days, it will help reduce inflammatory conditions. Boiled vegetables which are easily digestible and wheat chapattis may be added gradually to this diet. Later, rice dal, vegetable soup or buttermilk may be taken for lunch and an uncooked diet for dinner. The patient should avoid coffee, tea, and other stimulants as well as sugar, fried and refined foods.

Treatment through water plays an important role in overcoming vaginitis. The patient should be given enema with lukewarm neem water to cleanse the bowels and prevent constipation which increases the toxemic conditions, inflammation and infection in the genital organs. For general cleansing and elimination of purulent vaginal discharge, neem water vaginal douche at 35C - 40C followed by a cold douche will be highly beneficial.

In persistent cases, cold vaginal irritation provides relief. This treatment is best administered with a fountain syringe, containing water. The syringe should be placed two or three feet above the patient and water injected into the vagina. The patient should lie upon her back, with hips elevated and water should flow out of the vaginal canal.

A decoction of the herb chebulic myrobalan (harad) has proved very useful for vaginal irritation and inflammation. It should be used as an external douche to wash the vulval parts. When there is thick white discharge, washing the part with a decoction made with neem leaves and chebulic myrobalan fruits will greatly help.

A moderately prolonged cold hip bath accompanied with a hot foot bath is also helpful. Another mode of treatment considered beneficial is the wet girdle pack for about an hour. This helps reduce inflammation. Cold douche on the perineal region for 10 to 15 minutes and a mud pack on the abdomen for 10 minutes twice a day also help reduce inflammation.

After recovery, it is essential to adopt correct eating habits and hygienic living conditions. Proper rest and exercise are also important in the prevention and treatment of vaginitis.

SECTION IX

DISEASES OF ENDOCRINE SYSTEMS

CHAPTER 52

Diabetes

Many endocrine diseases may be seen occasionally in old age. The conditions of these diseases is an important factor because of their frequency. The most important of the endocrine disease commonly found in the elderly is diabetes.

Diabetes mellitus is a nutritional disorder, characterised by an abnormally elevated level of blood glucose and by the excretion of excess glucose in the urine. It results from an absolute or relative lack of insulin which leads to abnormalities in carbohydrates metabolism as well as in the metabolism of protein and fat.

The most commonly used screening tests are the determination of the fasting blood glucose level and the two-hour postprandial, that is, after a meal. The normal fasting blood sugar content is 80 to 120mg. per 100ml. of blood and this can go up to a level of 180mg. per 100ml. of blood two hours after meals. Anything above these norms can be termed diabetic levels.

Diabetes is extremely common in the elderly by any criteria. This is evident from the high blood sugar and abnormalities of the glucose tolerance test in old age. Diabetes in the elderly is often mild and most cases have their onset in old age. Clinical cases, that is those with symptoms or complications attributable to diabetes, outnumbered the cases which do not have any symptoms and are discovered by routine blood sugar determinations.

Symptoms

The word diabetes is derived from the Greek word meaning "to siphon, to pass through," and mellitus comes from the latin word "honey." Thus two characteristic symptoms, namely, copious urination and glucose in the urine give the name to the disease. The urine is of a pale colour, has an acidic reaction and sweetish colour.

A diabetic feels hungry and thirsty most of the time, does not put on weight, though he eats every now and then, and gets tired easily, both physically and mentally. He looks pale, may suffer from anaemia, constipation, intense itching around the genital organs, palpitations and general weakness. He feels drowsy and has a lower sex urge than a normal person.

Causes

Diabetes has been described by most biological doctors as a "prosperity" disease, primarily caused by systematic over eating and consequent obesity. Not only the overeating of sugar and refined carbohydrates, but also of proteins and fats, which are transformed into sugar, if taken in excess, is harmful and may result in diabetes. Too much food taxes the pancreas and eventually paralyses its normal activity.

Grief, worry and anxiety also have a deep influence on the metabolism and may cause sugar to appear in the urine. The diseases may be associated with some other grave organic disorders like cancer, tuberculosis and cerebral disease. Heredity is also a major factor in the development of the disease. It has been rightly said. "Heredity is like a cannon and obesity pulls the trigger."

Treatment

Any successful method for treatment of diabetes should aim at removal of the actual cause of the disease and building up of the whole health-level of the patient. Diet plays a vital role in such a treatment. The primary dietary consideration for a diabetes patient is that he should be a strict lactovegetarian and take a low-calorie, low-fat, alkaline diet of high quality natural foods. Fruits, nuts and vegetables, whole meal bread and dairy products form a good diet of the diabetic. These foods should be eaten in as dry a condition as possible to ensure thorough ensalivation during the first part of the process of digestion.

Cooked starchy foods should be avoided as in the process of cooking the cellulose envelopes of the starch granules burst and consequently, the starch is far too easily absorbed in the system. The excess absorbed has to be got rid of by the kidneys and appears as sugar in the urine. With raw starchy foods, however, the saliva and digestive juices in the small intestine regulate the quantities required to be changed into sugar for the body's needs. The unused and undigested portion of raw starchy foods does not become injurious to the system, as it does not readily ferment.

The diabetic should not be afraid to eat fresh fruits and vegetables which contain sugar and starch. Fresh fruits contain sugar fructose, which does not need insulin for its metabolism and is well tolerated by diabetics. Fats and oils should be taken sparingly, for they are apt to lower the tolerance for proteins and starches. Emphasis should be on raw foods as they stimulate and increase insulin production. For protein, home made cottage cheese, various forms of soured milk and nuts are best. The patient should avoid tea, coffee, cocoa, white flour, sugar and all the products from them, tinned fruits, refined cereals and alcoholic drinks. He should also avoid overeating and take four or five small meals a day rather than three large ones.

Among the several home remedies that have proved beneficial in controlling diabetes, perhaps the most important is the use of bitter gourd (Karela). Recent research by a team of British doctors have established that bitter gourd contains a hypoglycaemic or insulin-like principle, designated as 'plantinsulin,' which has been

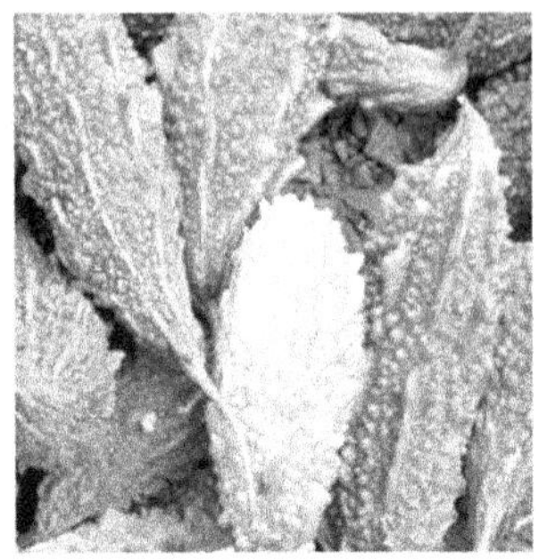

found valuable in lowering the blood and urine sugar levels. It should, therefore, be included liberally in the diet of the diabetic. For better results, the diabetic should take the juice of about four or five fruits every morning on an empty stomach. The seeds of bitter gourd can be added to food in a powdered form. Diabetics can also use bitter gourd in the form of decoction by boiling the pieces in water or in the form of dry powder.

Indian gooseberry (amla), with its high Vitamin C content, is considered valuable in diabetes. A tablespoon of its juice, mixed with half a cup of bitter gourd juice, taken daily for two months, will stimulate the islets of Langerhans i.e. the isolated group of cells that secrete the hormone insulin. It thus reduces the blood sugar in diabetes.

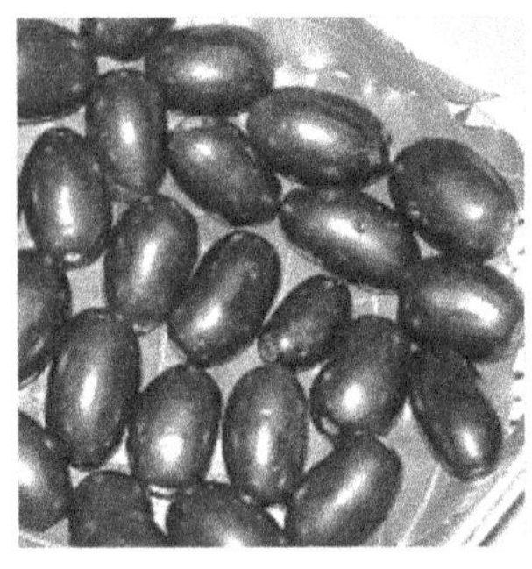

Jambul fruit (Jamun) is another effective home remedy. It is regarded in traditional medicine as a specific against diabetes because of its effect on the pancreas. The fruits as such, the seeds and fruit juice are all useful in the treatment of this disease. The seeds contain in glucoside 'jamboline' which is believed to have the power to check the pathological conversion of starch into sugar in cases of increased production of glucose. They should be dried and powdered. This powder should be taken mixed in milk, curd or water.

The inner bark of the jambul tree is also used in the treatment of diabetes. The bark is dried and burnt. It will produce an ash of white colour. This ash should be pestled in mortar, strained and bottled. The diabetic patient should be given 10 grams of this ash on an empty stomach with water in the morning and 20 grams each time in the afternoon and in the evening after an hour of taking meals.

According to Dr. Joe Shelby Riley, a well-known expert in nutrition, "Grapefruit (Chakotra) is a splendid thing in the food of diabetic patient. If grapefruits were eaten more liberally, there would be much less diabetes. If you have sugar, use three grapefruits three times a day. If you do not have sugar, but a tendency towards it and want to prevent it, use three a day."

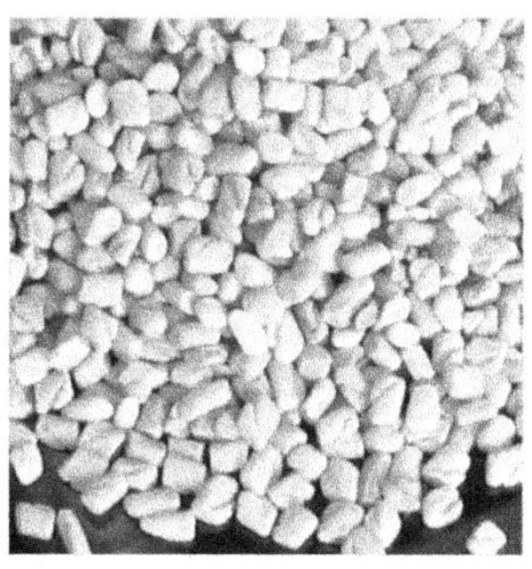

The seeds of fenugreek (Methi) have been found effective in the treatment of diabetes. According to a recent report brought out by Indian Council of Medical Research, fenugreek seeds, when given in varying doses of 25 grams to 100 grams daily, diminish reactive hyperglycemia in diabetic patients. Levels of glucose, serum cholesterol and tryglycerides were also significantly reduced in the diabetes patients when the seeds were consumed.

Experiments have shown that the intake of water extract of bengal gram (Chana) enhances the utilization of glucose in both the diabetic and the normal persons. Tests were conducted at CFITRI Laboratories in Mysore, on a chronic diabetes patient whose insulin requirements was of the order of 40 units a day. When kept on a diet which included liberal supplements of Bengal gram extract, the condition of the patient improved considerably and his insulin requirement was reduced to about 20 units per day. Diabetes patients who are on a prescribed diet which does not severely restrict the intake of carbohydrates, but includes liberal amounts of Bengal gram extract, have shown considerable improvement in their fasting blood sugar levels, glucose tolerance, urinary excretion of sugar and general condition.

The tender leaves of the mango tree are considered useful in diabetes. An infusion is prepared from fresh leaves by soaking them overnight and squeezing them well in water in the morning. This filtrate should be taken every morning to control early diabetes. In the alternative, the leaves should be dried in the shade, powdered and preserved for use when necessary. Half a teaspoon of this powder should be taken twice a day.

The juice of Margosa leaves is helpful in controlling diabetes. One tablespoon (5 ml) of this juice should be taken early in the morning on an empty stomach for this purpose. This treatment should be continued for 3 months. In the alternative, 10 leaves should be chewed daily in the morning.

Besides bitter gourd, certain other vegetables have been found useful in diabetes. These include string beans, cucumbers, onion and garlic. String bean pod tea is an excellent natural substitute for insulin and valuable in diabetes. Cucumbers contain a hormone needed by the cells of the pancreas for producing insulin. Onions and garlic have proved beneficial in reducing blood sugar in diabetes.

Exercise is also an important factor in the treatment of diabetes. Light games, jogging and swimming are helpful. Yogic asanas such as bhujangasana, halasana, shalbhasana, dhanurasana, paschimottanasana, sarvangasana and shavasana, yogic kriyas like jalaneti, and kunjal, and pranayamas such as kapalbahati, anulomaviloma and ujjayi will also be beneficial.

Hydrotherapy forms an important part of the treatment. The colon should be thoroughly cleansed daily with warm water enema, until the bowel discharge assumes normal characteristics. Bathing in cold water greatly increases the circulation and enhances the capacity of the muscles to utilise sugar.

The diabetic patient should eliminate minor worries from his daily life. He must endeavour to be more easy-going and should not get unduly worked up by the stress and strain of life.

CHAPTER 53

Thyroid Disease

The thyroid gland is the best known of the ductless glands. It lies in the neck in front of the windpipe, just below the Adam's apple. Through its secretions, thyroxin, it regulates the day-to-day activities, maintains homeostasis through the periods of stress and strain and provides fine balance to the regulatory systems of the body. No part of the body seems to escape its influence.

Dr. Louis Berman, a famous endocrinologist, has described the vital functions of thyroid glands as follows: "Without the thyroid there can be no complexity of thought, no learning, no education, no habit formation, no responsive energy for situations as well as no physical unfolding of faculty and function. No reproduction of kind, with no sign of adolescence at the expected age and no exhibition of sex tendencies thereafter."

The normal thyroid gland does not enlarge with age. There is decrease in follicular size and increase in connective tissue. These normal age-related changes, together with an increased frequency of pathological nodules, give the appearance of thyroid enlargement.

Women are more prone to thyroid disease. They are especially likely to develop a sluggish thyroid after middle age. The disease is more common in women who are over worked and who do not get sufficient rest and relaxation. The period in older women's life, when she is more likely to be affected by this disease, is at the menopause and thereafter, or when there is any extra physical strain on the body.

Thyroid disease assumes various forms, the most frequent being hypothyroidism, also known as myxedema, and hyperthyroidism, also known as thyrotoxicosis or exopthalmic goitre. Hypothyroidism results from the withering or atrophy of the thyroid gland. Hyperthyroidism is a serious condition of the body, which results from overactivity of the thyroid gland.

Hypothyroidism is a common condition in the elderly. It is second only to diabetes as an endocrine disorder in old age. Hyperthyroidism, after 60 years of age, comprises about one-third to one-half of all cases. The annual incidence is about 0.98 per 1000, which is seven times the frequency in the younger population.

Symptoms

In hypothyroidism, the basal metabolism decreases below normal, with the result the patient tends to be slow in his movements. He is susceptible to cold, suffers from constipation and puts on weight. His hair become dry, scaly and thickened. There may be puffiness in his face, especially around his eyes. The pulse is slow and the patient often complains of vague pains in the back and stiffness in the joints.

The patient with hyperthyroidism is usually nervous, weak, sensitive to heat, sweats frequently, is overactive and often underweight. There may be slight tremor in the fingers and palpitation of the heart. In many cases, there may be bulging of the eyes and passing of excessive quantities of urine. The heart is overactive and usually enlarged. The pulse rate is rapid and may be irregular.

Causes

The main cause of hypothyroidism is insufficient production

of thyroid hormone. Other causes of this disease are some pituitary deficiency and inborn error of the thyroid gland. The change usually comes gradually. The main cause of hyperthyroidism is the excess amounts of thyroid hormone produced by the overactive gland. This raises the metabolic rate of the body. Another important cause of this disease is physical or emotional stress. Heredity also plays a role and the disease seems to run in families.

The real cause of thyroid disease, however, is wrong feeding habits over a long period and faulty style of living, together with suppressive medical treatment of other diseases in the past. The thyroid gland plays an important role in destroying toxic matter generated in the intestines as a result of the putrefaction of animal protein material, like meat, fish, eggs, cheese and milk. The thyroid gland will be overworked when excessive quantities of these foods are consumed, resulting in the clogging of the intestinal tract with toxic matter. The overworking of the thyroid gland is further complicated by wrong living habits and excessive emotionalism, both of which weaken the system.

Treatment

The only real treatment for thyroid disease, whether hypothyroidism, hyperthyroidism or any other condition of thyroid gland, is cleansing of the system and adoption of a rational diet thereafter, combined with adequate rest and relaxation. To begin with, juices of fruits such as orange, apple, pineapple, and grapes may be taken every two or three hours from 8 a.m. to 8 p.m. for five days. The bowels should be cleaned daily with lukewarm water.

After the juice fast, the patient may spend further three days on fruits and milk, taking three meals a day of juicy fruits such as apple, pineapple, grapes, papaya, with a glass of milk, at five hourly intervals. Thereafter, the patient may adopt a well-balanced diet consisting of seeds, nuts and grains, vegetables and fruits.

The patient should take plenty of rest and spend a day in bed every week for the first two months of the treatment. More and more exercise should be taken after the symptoms subside.

The appetite of the thyroid patient is usually very large and the weight reduction cannot be prevented for some time. This is because until the heart beat slows down and the tremors stop, there will be incomplete assimilation of food. But as soon as the balance is restored, weight will slowly increase. To help the absorption of food, a narrow waist compress and, later, a neck compress should be worn for five nights a week. As weight increases, the almost constant hunger will gradually disappear, on no account should any stimulants be administered to create an appetite.

Certain foods and fluids are extremely injurious for thyroid patients and should be avoided by them. These include white flour products, white sugar, fresh foods, fried or greasy foods, preserves, condiments, tea, coffee and alcohol.

No drugs should be taken as they cause irritation in the tissues. Iodine is undoubtedly most helpful in many cases, but it should be introduced in organic form. All foods containing iodine should be taken liberally. These are asparagus, cabbage, garlic, onion, oats, pineapple, whole rice, tomatoes, watercress and strawberries.

Great care must be taken never to allow the body to become exhausted and any irritation likely to cause emotional upset should be avoided. The cure of thyroid disease is not a speedy one and there is often a recurrence of symptoms but these should gradually become less pronounced. Strict adherence to diet is essential for complete cure.

Half the daily intake of food should consist of fresh fruits and vegetables and the starch element should be confined to whole wheat products and potatoes. Potatoes are the most valuable form of starch. They should preferably be taken with their jackets. The protein foods should be confined to cheese, peas, beans lentils and nuts. All fresh proteins must be avoided.

The diet outlined here should be strictly adhered to for a year and the compresses on neck and waist applied for five consecutive nights in a week for two months and discontinued for one month. Water treatments should be taken to increase skin elimination. Application of sponge to the entire body before retiring and a cold sponge on rising will be very helpful. It is most important that the bowels are kept working efficiently to avoid danger of a toxic condition of the blood arising from that source.

All efforts should be made to prevent emotional stress. There may be slight recurrence of this extremely nervous complain for some time, but the attacks will become less severe and of shorter duration as the treatment progresses. Above all, there must be no lessening of the patient's efforts to help himself because success can only be attained by assiduous efforts.

SECTION X

OTHER DISEASES

CHAPTER 54

Anaemia

Anaemia may be described as a condition in which there is a decrease in the quantity of haemoglobin, in the number of red cells, in the volume of packed cells, or in a combination of these. The World Health Organisation defines it as a condition in which haemoglobin concentration, or the number of red blood cells, is below the level which is normal for a given individual.

Anaemia is widely prevalent in old age and its incidence increases with advancing age. Studies show that approximately six to ten per cent of females above the age of 60 are at moderate risk of anaemia, which is similar to the risk found in middle aged females. In men above the age of 60, approximately 15 per cent are at moderate risk of anaemia, which is much higher than that found in younger males. Further studies indicate that only a small proportion of males and females above the age of 60 are at high risk of anaemia. The incidence of this disease in both males and females is significantly higher in the eighth decade than in the seventh, with an even higher incidence in elderly persons aged over 80.

Anaemia is particularly common in old people who are sick. It is also not rare in apparently healthy old people. Evidence, however, shows that the incidence of anaemia is much higher in sick and neglected elderly people than in the healthy, presumably due to dietary deficiency.

Nearly half of the blood flowing in our veins and arteries consists of red blood cells which carry oxygen to the tissues. Approximately, one trillion (100 million) new blood cells are formed daily in the bone marrow. The raw materials required in the production of these cells are iron, proteins and vitamins, especially folic acid and B12. Of these, iron and proteins are essential in building up the red colouring matter, called haemoglobin.

Red cells live approximately 120 days and are being destroyed and replaced daily. Each person should have 100 per cent of haemoglobin or about 15 grams to 100 ml of blood, and a blood count of 5 million red cells per millimeter. A drop in the haemoglobin content results in anaemia.

The level of 12g/100ml is probably the best criterion to describe anaemia in old age. Moderate risk of anaemia is defined as a value between 12 and 14g/100ml for males and between 10 to 12g/100ml for females. High risk of anaemia is indicated by a value below 12g/100ml for males and 10g/100ml for females.

Symptoms

The patient usually complains of weakness, easy fatigue, lack of energy and dizziness. Other symptoms include a haggard look, premature wrinkles, dull and tired looking eyes, poor memory, shortness of breath on exertion, headache, slow healing of wounds, palpitation of heart and mental depression. The skin and mucous membranes look pale, and nails appear brittle and there may be sores at the corners of the mouth.

The subtle signs and symptoms of anaemia are more difficult to detect in the elderly than in young adults. The condition itself may be a symptom of an underlying disease like tumour, ulcer, hiatus, hernia, bleeding piles, infection and other disease. In case of decrease in haemoglobin, the important manifestations in the old are palpitation, breathlessness, postural hypotension, giddiness and the onset of congestive cardiac failure.

Causes

Low formation of red blood cells in the bone marrow, either due to defects in the bone marrow or to an inadequate intake of iron, vitamin and protein, is one of the main causes of anaemia. Another important cause is heavy loss of blood due to injury and other conditions. Other causes include lack of digestive acid or hydrochloric acid needed for digestion of iron and proteins and emotional strain, anxiety and worry which interferes with the manufacture of hydrochloric acid in the body. Intestinal parasites or worms are yet other little known causes of anaemia. They feed on the supply of blood as well as vitamins.

Nutritional factors play an important role in causing anaemia in the elderly. Old people are vulnerable to dietary inadequacies and many elderly persons have blood and tissue levels of nutrients which are below the normal levels of younger age groups. Folic acid deficiency is common in the elderly, but anaemia solely due to folic acid deficiency is not common. Dietary deficiency of Vitamin B12 is seen in vegans but elderly vegans are relatively rare.

Treatment

Diet is of utmost importance in the treatment of anaemia. Refined foods like white bread, polished rice, sugar and desserts rob the body of the much needed iron. Iron should always be taken in its natural organic form in food as the use of inorganic iron can prove hazardous. It may cause destruction of protective vitamins and unsaturated fatty acids, serious liver damage, miscarriage during pregnancy and delayed or premature birth in younger females.

The diet should be predominantly alkaline. The emphasis should be on raw fruits and vegetables which are rich in iron. Iron-rich vegetables are spinach, green onions, squash, carrots, radishes, beets, celery, yams, tomatoes and potatoes (with jackets). Fruits which are rich in iron are bananas, apples, dark grapes, apricots, plums, raisins and strawberries. Bananas are particularly beneficial as they also contain, besides easily assimilable iron, folic acid and B12, both of which are extremely useful in the treatment of anaemia.

Other iron-rich foods are whole wheat, brown rice, beans, soyabeans, sunflower seeds, crude blackstrap molasses, eggs and honey. Honey is also rich in copper which helps in iron absorption. The diet should also be adequate in proteins of high biological value such as milk, home-made cottage cheese and eggs.

Vitamin B12 is a must for preventing or curing anaemia. This vitamin is usually found in animal protein especially in organic meats like kidney and liver. A heavy meat diet is often associated with a high haemoglobin and high red cell count, but it has its disadvantages. One cause of anaemia is intestinal putrefaction, which is primarily brought on by a high meat diet. Moreover, all meat are becoming increasingly dangerous due to widespread diseases in animal kingdom. There are, however, other equally good sources of Vitamin B12 such as dairy products, like milk, eggs, cheese and peanuts. Wheat germ and soyabean also contain some B12. Vegetarians should include adequate amount of milk, milk products and eggs in their diet.

For prevention of anaemia, it is essential to take the entire B complex range which includes B12, as well as the natural foods mentioned above. Eating lacto-avo products, which are complete proteins and which also contain Vitamin B12, is good insurance against the disease. A liberal intake of ascorbic acid is also necessary to facilitate absorption of iron. At least two helpings of citrus fruits and other ascorbic-rich foods should be taken daily.

Mention must be made of beets (chukandar) which are extremely important in curing anaemia. Beet juice contains potassium, phosphorous, calcium, sulphur, iodine, iron, copper, carbohydrates, protein, fat, Vitamin B1, B2, niacin B6, C and Vitamin P. With its high iron content, beet juice regenerates and reactivates the red blood cells, supplies the body with fresh oxygen and helps the normal function of vesicular breathing. According to Dr. Firitz Keitel of Germany. "The juice of red beet strengthens the body's power of resistance and has proved to be an excellent remedy for anaemia, especially for children and teenagers, where other blood forming remedies have failed."

Lettuce (salad ka patta) is another effective remedy for this disease. It contains considerable amount of iron and supplies a good form of vegetable haemoglobin. It can, therefore, be used as a good tonic food for anaemia. The iron obtained in this way is absorbed by the body to a much greater degree than the inorganic iron tonic.

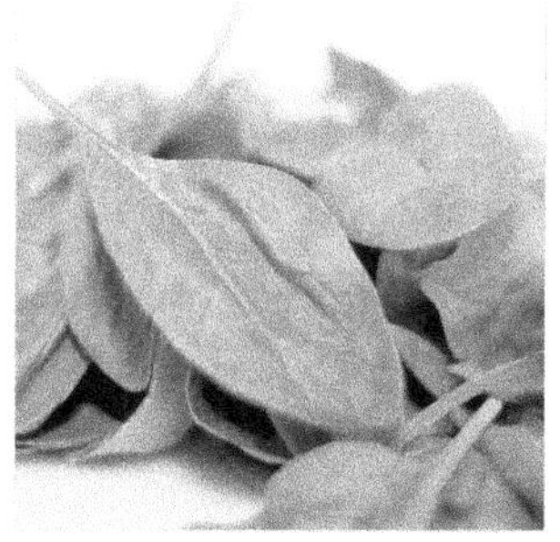

The use of spinach (Palak) is valuable in anaemia. It is a rich source of high grade iron. After its absorption in the system, the formation of haemoglobin and red blood cells takes place. It is thus beneficial in building up the blood and in the prevention and treatment of anaemia.

Soyabean (bhat), being rich in iron, has proved beneficial in the treatment of anaemia. As, the anaemia patients suffer from weak digestion, it should be given to them in a very light form, preferably in the form of milk, which may be easily digested.

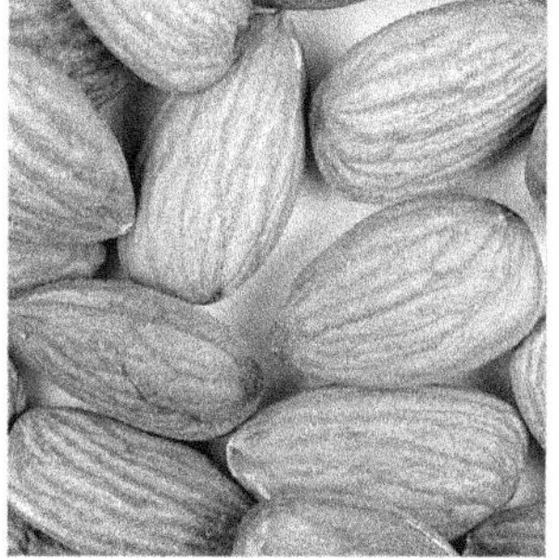

Almond (badam) is another effective remedy for anaemia. It contains copper in organic form at the rate of 1.15 mg. per 100 grams. The copper along with iron and vitamins, acts as a catalyst in the synthesis of blood haemoglobin. This dry fruit is therefore a useful remedy for anaemia. Black sesame seeds (Til), as a rich source of iron, are also valuable in anaemia. An emulsion of the seeds is prepared by grinding and straining them after soaking them in warm water for a couple of hours. This emulsion, mixed with a cup of milk and sweetened with jaggery, should be given to patients suffering from this disease.

An anaemic person should commence the dietary treatment by an exclusive fresh fruit diet for about five days. During this period, he should take three meals of fresh juicy fruits at five hourly intervals. This may be followed by fruit and milk diet for about 15 days. In this regimen, the meals are exactly the same as for all-fruit diet, but with milk added to each fruit meal. The patient may begin with one litre of milk the first day and increase by 250 ml daily upto 2 litres a day, depending on how the milk agrees. After the fruit and milk diet, the patient may gradually embark upon a well-balanced diet based on three basic food groups, namely (i) seeds, nuts and grains (ii) vegetables and (iii) fruits.

A cold water bath is among the most valuable curative measures in anaemia. The patient should be given carefully graduated cold baths twice daily. Cold friction, hot epsom salt bath for 5 to 10 minutes once a week are also recommended. Full sun baths are especially beneficial as sunlight stimulates the production of red cells. Deep breathing and light exercise like walking and simple yoga asanas should be undertaken to tone up the system. Sarvangsana, paschimottanasana, uttanapadasana and shavasana are recommended. Massage also helps to keep the blood level high.

CHAPTER 55

Cancer

The word 'Cancer' comes from the latin 'Carcinoma' meaning crab. It is the most dreaded disease and refers to all malignant tumours caused by the abnormal growth of a body cell or a group of cells. It is today the second largest killer in the world, next only to heart ailments. The term covers more than 20 diseases.

There is a close relationship between cancer and ageing. In the United States, over one-half of all cancers occur in 11 per cent of the population over the age of 65. At the age of 25, the probability of developing cancer within five years is one in 700, while at the age of 65, it is one in 14. The peak incidence and mortality of cancer is in the 60-75 age range.

Although deaths attributable to cancer decrease from 30 per cent at age 50 to 10 per cent or less at age 85, this is largely due to the rapid increase in death due to other causes with advancing age, and not due to non-prevalence of cancer. Despite the marked increase in cardiovascular related deaths with age, cancer remains the second leading cause of death in those over 65.

There are billions of cells in the body which, under normal circumstances, develop in a well-organised pattern for the growth of the body and the repair of damaged tissues. When cancer sets in, a group of cells start multiplying suddenly in a haphazard manner and form a lump or tumour. Cancer can spread very rapidly and eventually prove fatal, if not treated properly and in time.

Sex does not affect the incidence of the disease. It, however, affects the site of growth. In men, cancer is usually found in the intestines, the prostate and the lungs. In women, it occurs mostly in the breast tissues, uterus, gallbladder and thyroid.

Symptoms

The symptoms of cancer vary according to the site of the growth. The American Cancer Society has prescribed seven signs or danger signals in general which may indicate the presence of cancer. These are; a sore that does not heal; change in bowel or bladder habits; unusual bleeding or discharge; thickening or lump in breast or elsewhere; indigestion or difficulty in swallowing; obvious change in wart or mole and persistent and nagging cough or hoarseness. Other symptoms may include unexplained loss of weight, particularly in older people, change in skin colour and changes in the menstrual periods, especially bleeding between periods.

Cancers have a latency period varying from 5 to 40 years between the initial exposure to a carcinogen and the time the symptoms appear. In a large number of cases, either trivial symptoms are noted or there are none at all. One has, therefore to be vigilant to recognise the first sign of the disease. The best way of diagnosing cancer is through a process called 'biopsy', in which a piece of suspect tissue is examined and tested under a microscope.

Causes

The prime cause of cancer is not known. Certain cancer causing substances, known as carcinogens, however, increase the chances of getting the disease. About 80 per cent of cancers are caused by environmental factors. 40 per cent of male cancers in India are linked with tobacco, a known cancer-causing agent. The consumption of paan, betelnut, tobacco and slaked lime has been linked with cancer of the tongue, lips, mouth and throat.

Cigarette and beedi smoking and hukka puffing are linked with lung and throat cancers. Heavy consumption of alcoholic drinks can cause oesophagal, stomach and liver cancers. Occupational exposure to industrial pollutants such as asbestos, nickel, tar, soot and high doses of X-Rays can lead to skin and lung cancers and leukaemia.

Other factors contributing to cancer are viral infections, trauma, hormone imbalance and malnutrition. Many well-known biologists and naturopaths believe that a faulty diet is the root cause of cancer. Investigations indicate that the cancer incidence is in direct proportion to the amount of animal protein, particularly meat, in the diet. Dr. Willard J Visek, a renowned research scientist, explained recently a link between excessive meat-eating and cancer. According to him, the villain is ammonia, the carcinogenic by-product of meat digestion.

Treatment

The effective treatment of cancer consists of a complete change in diet, besides total elimination of all environmental sources of carcinogens, such as smoking and carcinogenic chemicals in air, water and food. As a first step, the patient should cleanse the system by thoroughly relieving constipation and making all the organs of elimination — the skin, lungs, liver, kidneys and bowels — active. Warm water enema should be used to cleanse the colon. For the first four or five days, the patient should take only juicy fruits like orange, grapefruit, lemon, apple, peach, pear, pineapple and grapes. Vegetable juices are also useful, especially carrot and tomato juices.

After an exclusive fruit diet, the patient may be given a nourishing alkaline-based diet. It should consist of 100 per cent natural foods, with emphasis on fresh raw fruits and vegetables, particularly carrots, green leafy vegetables, cabbage, onion, garlic, cucumber, beets and tomatoes. A minimum requirement of high quality protein, mostly from vegetable spices such as almonds, millet, sesame seeds, sprouted seeds and grains, may be added to this diet.

Diet

Diet is now considered a major factor in the prevention and treatment of cancer. According to the American National Cancer Institute about one-third of the cancers are linked to diet. Thus, right choices of foods can help prevent a majority of new cancer cases and deaths from cancer.

Cancer usually develops over a long period. Latest research shows that what one eats may interfere with cancer process at many stages, from conception to growth and spread of the cancer. Foods can block the chemical activation which normally initiates cancer. Antioxidants, including vitamins can eradicate carcinogens and can even repair some of the cellular damage caused by them. Cancers which are in the process of growth can also be prevented from further spreading by foods. Even in advanced cases, the right foods can prolong the patient's life.

Researches conducted in ascertaining links between diet and cancer since 1970 have now conclusively proved that fruits and vegetables can serve as antidote to cancer. According to Dr. Peter Greenwald, Director of the Division of Cancer Prevention and Control at the American National Cancer Institute: "The more fruits and vegetables people eat, the less likely they are to get cancer." Some studies indicate that eating fruit twice a day instead of less than three times a week, cut the risk of lung cancer 75 per cent, even in smokers.

The normal servings of fruits and vegetables are two fruits and three vegetables a day. Adding more fruits and vegetables to these servings can reduce the risk of cancer.

The plant foods which are considered to possess anti-cancer properties by the American National Cancer Institute include vegetables like garlic, cabbage, tomato, soya beans, ginger, carrot, celery, onion, broccoli, cauliflower, brussels sprouts and cucumber; citrus fruits like orange, grapefruit, lemon and lime; other foods like turmeric, whole wheat, brown rice, barely and berries; and herbs like rosemary, sage, thyme, chives and basil.

A Nobel Prize winner of the University of Pennsylvania Medical School, Dr. Otto Meyerhof, spoke of the evidence connecting the excessive consumption of sugar with cancer by calling attention to "the appetite of tumors for sugar." He suggested that the growth of cancerous tissue might possibly be stopped if biochemists could find a way of curing this appetite.

Recent researches have shown that certain vitamins can be successfully employed in the fight against cancer and that they can increase the life expectancy of some terminal cancer patients. According to recent Swedish studies, Vitamin C in large doses can be an effective prophylactic agent against cancer. Noted Japanese scientist Dr. Fukumi Morishige and his colleague who have been examining the healing potential of Vitamin C for many years, have found that mixture of Vitamin C and copper compound has lethal effects on cancer.

According to several studies, Vitamin A exerts an inhibiting effect on carcinogenesis. It is one of the most important aids to the body's defence system to fight and prevent cancer. A recent British study found that cancer rates dropped by 40 per cent in men with the most blood beta carotene (a precursor of Vitamin A), compared with those with the least. Other research has found that those with higher levels of folic acid (found in green vegetable) and lycopene (a tomato compound) are much less vulnerable to all cancers, in particular of the lung, cervix and pancreas.

Johanna Brandt, the author of the book *The Grape Cure*, has advocated an exclusive grape diet for the treatment of cancer. She discovered this mode of cure in 1920, while experimenting on herself by fasting and dieting alternately in the course of her nine-year battle with cancer. She claimed to have cured herself by this mode of treatment. She recommends fast for two or three days so as to prepare the system for the change of diet.

Dr. Ann Wigmore of Boston, U.S.A., the well-known naturopath and pioneer in the field of living food nutrition, has been testing the effect of a drink made of fresh wheatgrass in the treatment of leukaemia. She claims to have cured several cases of this disease by this method. Dr. Wigmore points our that by furnishing the body with live minerals, vitamins, trace elements and chlorophyll through wheatgrass juice, it may be able to repair itself.

The use of margosa (neem) leaves are considered beneficial as supportive treatment of cancer, according to Ayurveda. From the point of view of this system of medicine, the blood gets toxicated and body heat increases in this disease. Margosa leaves help in purifying the blood and in reducing body heat. The patient Should therefore chew 10-12 margosa leaves daily in the morning.

Prevention

It is, however, more important to prevent the disease than treat it, as measures to treat the disease bring only temporary result in view of the poor survival rate after the use of such treatment.

The best way to prevent cancer is to build up the body's defences through excellent nutrition. The tissues, cells and organs should be kept in such a healthy state that cancer cannot take hold. This can be achieved by completely avoiding all refined, synthetic and processed foods as also white flour, enriched fortified foods, white sugar and foods with chemical additives. The foods which build up the body are natural, whole foods, raw vegetables and fruits, protein from vegetable sources, milk, whole grains and vitamins and minerals in their natural form.

The other preventive measures are plenty of rest, complete freedom from worries and mental stress and plenty of fresh, pure air.

CHAPTER 56

High Blood Cholesterol

High blood cholesterol, known as hypercholesterolemia in medical parlance, refers to an increase in the cholesterol in blood above the normal level. It is a major factor in coronary artery disease. A person with a high blood cholesterol is regarded as a potential candidate for heart attack, a stroke or high blood pressure.

Cholesterol is a yellow fatty substance and a principal ingredient in the digestive juice bile, in the fatty sheaths that insulate nerves and in sex hormones, namely estrogen and androgen. It performs several functions such as transportation of fat, providing defence mechanism, protecting red blood cells and muscular membrane of the body.

Most of the cholesterol found in the body is produced in the liver. However, about 20 to 30 per cent generally comes from the foods we eat. Some cholesterol is also secreted into the intestinal tract in bile and becomes mixed with the dietary cholesterol. The percentage of ingested cholesterol absorbed seems to average 40 to 50 per cent of the intake.

The amount of cholesterol is measured in milligrams per 100 ml of blood. Normal level of cholesterol varies between 150-250 mg per 100 ml. Persons with atherosclerosis have uniformly high blood cholesterol, usually above 250 mg per 100 ml.

In blood, cholesterol is bound to certain proteins — lipoproteins which have an affinity for blood fats, known as lipids. There are two main types of lipoproteins, a low density one (LDL) and a high density one (HDL). The low density lipoprotein is the one which is considered harmful and is associated with cholesterol deposits in blood vessels. The higher the ratio of LDL to the total cholesterol, the greater will be the risk of the arterial damage and heart disease. The HDL on the other hand plays a salutary role by helping remove cholesterol from circulation and thereby reduce the risk of heart disease.

Cholesterol has been the subject of extensive study by researchers since 1769, when French Chemist, Poluteir de la Salle purified the soapy-looking yellowish substance. The results of the most comprehensive research study, commissioned by the National Heart and Lung Institute of the U.S.A., were announced in 1985. The 10-year study, considered most elaborate and most extensive research project in medical history, indicates that heart disease is directly linked to the level of cholesterol in the blood and that lowering cholesterol level significantly reduces the incidence of heart attacks by two per cent.

The relative contributions of low density lipoproteins (LDL) to high density lipoproteins (HDL) to total serum cholesterol changes with age. This change makes it difficult to predict the contribution of total serum cholesterol to coronary heart disease in the elderly. The association of high blood cholesterol to coronary heart disease is well established in the younger age group. Experts doubt whether this data is valid for elderly persons also, and whether the reduction in serum cholesterol could arrest the progression of coronary atherosclerosis in old age.

However, the reduction of cholesterol level in the elderly has assumed great significance in recent years with latest studies conducted at National Heart and Lung Institute. These studies have proved that high blood cholesterol constitutes a risk factor in atherosclerosis in the elderly and that a drastic reduction in the blood cholesterol could lead to its retardation in old age. Age itself being a major risk factor for coronary heart disease, treatment of high blood cholesterol is of utmost importance in the elderly, as it may lead to a greater reduction in relative risk than in younger patients.

Causes

Hypercholesterolemia is mainly a digestive problem caused by rich foods such as fried foods, excessive consumption of milk and its products like ghee, butter and cream, white flour, sugar, cakes, pastries, biscuits, cheese, ice-cream as well as non-vegetarian foods like meat, fish and eggs. Other causes of increase in cholesterol are irregularity in habits, smoking and drinking alcohol.

Stress has been found to be a major cause of increased level of cholesterol. Adrenaline and cortisone are both released in the body under stress. This, in turn, produces a fat metabolising reaction. Adrenal glands of executive–type aggressive persons produce more adrenaline than the easy going men. Consequently, they suffer six to eight times more heart attacks than the relaxed men.

Treatment

To reduce the risk of heart disease, it is essential to lower the level of LDL and increase the level of HDL cholesterol. This can be achieved by improving the diet and changing the life style. Diet is the most important factor. As a first step, foods rich in cholesterol and saturated fats, which lead to increase in LDL level, should be reduced to the minimum. Cholesterol-rich foods are eggs, virtually all foods of animal origin as well as two vegetable oils, namely coconut and palm, are high in saturated fats and these should be replaced by polyunsaturated fats such as corn, safflower, soyabeans and sesame oils which tend to lower the level of LDL. There are mono saturated fats such as olive and peanut oils which have more or less neutral effect on the LDL level.

The American Heart Association recommends that men should restrict themselves to 300 mg of cholesterol a day and women to 275 mg. It also prescribes that fat should not make up more than 30 per cent of the diet and not more than one-third of this should be saturated. The Association, however, urges somewhat strict regimen for those who already have elevated levels of cholesterol.

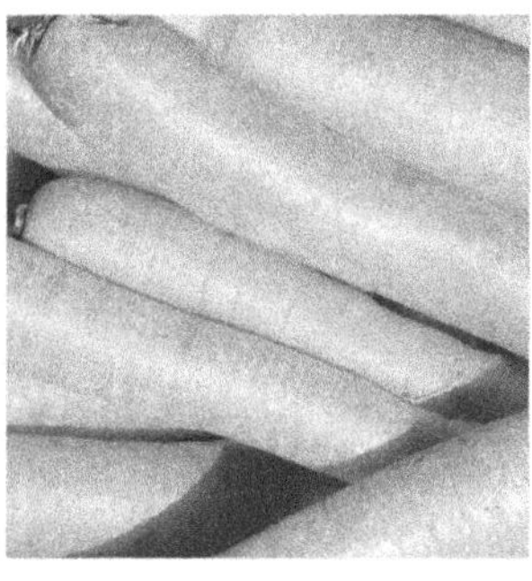

The amount of fibre in the diet also influences the cholesterol levels and LDL cholesterol can be lowered by taking diets rich in fibres. The most significant sources of dietary fibre are unprocessed wheat bran, whole cereals such as wheat, rice, barley, rye; legumes such as potato, carrot, beet and turnips; fruits like mango and guava and leafy vegetable such as cabbage, lady's finger, lettuce and celery. Oat bran are specially beneficial in lowering LDL cholesterol.

Lecithin, also a fatty food substance and the most abundant of the phospholipids, is highly beneficial in case of increase in cholesterol level. It has the ability to break up cholesterol into small particles which can be easily handled by the system. With sufficient intake of lecithin, cholesterol cannot build up against the walls of the arteries and veins. It also increases the production of bile acids made from cholesterol, thereby reducing its amount in the blood. Egg yolk, vegetable oils, whole grain cereals, soyabeans and unpasturised milk are rich sources of lecithin. The cells of the body are also capable of synthesizing it as needed, if several of the B Vitamins are present.

Diets high in Vitamin B6, choline and inositol supplied by wheat germ, yeast or B Vitamin extracted from bran have been particularly effective in reducing blood cholesterol. Sometimes, Vitamin E elevates blood lecithin and reduces cholesterol presumably by preventing the essential fatty acids from being destroyed by oxygen.

Several studies suggest that calcium can help lower blood cholesterol. In a study led by Dr. Margo Denke at the University of Texas, 13 men with high blood cholesterol levels were given a low-calcium diet (410 mg of calcium daily) for 10 days, and had their cholesterol levels checked. Then, for another 10 days, they were given a fortified diet that supplied 2200 mg of calcium daily. The result was that the high calcium regimen reduced their levels of total cholesterol by six per cent and slashed 'bad' LDL cholesterol by 11 per cent. However, 'good' HDL Cholesterol levels remain the same.

The sunflower (suryamukhi) seeds are valuable in high blood cholesterol. They contain substantial quantity of linoleic acid which is the fat helpful in reducing cholesterol deposits on the walls of arteries. Substituting sunflower seeds for some of the solid fats like butter and cream will, therefore, lead to great improvement in health.

Regular drinking of a decoction of coriander (dhaniya) seeds helps lower blood cholesterol. It is a good diuretic and helps stimulates the kidneys. It is prepared by boiling the dry seeds and straining the decoction after cooling.

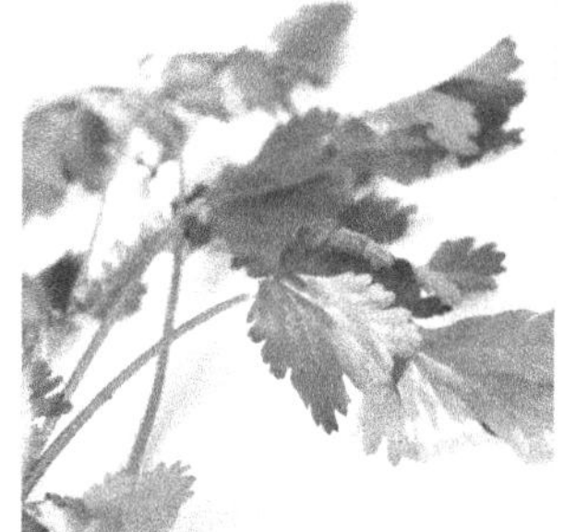

The herb ispaghula (ishabgul) has been found beneficial in the treatment of high cholesterol level. The embryo oil of the seeds of this plant should be given for lowering blood cholesterol. It contains 50 per cent linoleic acid. This oil is more active than safflower oil.

Persons with high blood cholesterol level should drink at least eight to 10 glasses of water every day as copious drinking of water stimulates the excretory activity of the skin and kidneys. This, in turn, facilitates elimination of excessive cholesterol from the system.

Regular exercise also plays an important role in lowering LDL cholesterol and in raising the level of protective HDL. It also promotes circulation and helps maintain the blood flow to every part of the body. Jogging or brisk walking, swimming, bicycling and playing badminton are excellent forms of exercise.

Yogasanas are beneficial as they help increase perspiratory activity and stimulate sebaceous glands to effectively secrete accumulated or excess cholesterol from the muscular tissue. Asanas like shalabhasana, padmasana and vajrasana are useful in lowering blood cholesterol by increasing systemic activity.

Hydrotherapy can be successfully employed in reducing excess cholesterol. Cold hip baths for 10 minutes taken twice every day have proved beneficial. Steam baths are also helpful except in patients suffering from hypertension and other circulatory disorders. Mudpacks, applied over the abdomen improve digestion and assimilation. They improve the functioning of the liver and other digestive organs and activate kidneys and the intestines to promote better excretion. The procedure for the various baths and mud packs has been explained in the Appendix.

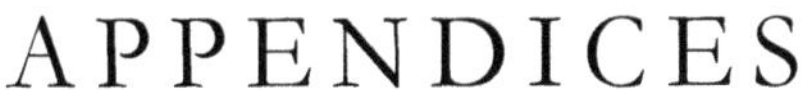

APPENDICES

Chart Showing the Common Foods with Acid and Alkaline Ash

Food Leaving an Acid Ash

Barley	Eggs
Bananas (unripe)	Grain Foods
Beans	Lentils
Bread	Meats
Cereals	Nuts except almonds
Cakes	Oatmeal
Chicken	Peas
Confection	Rice
Cheese	Sugar
Chocolate	Tea
Coffee	

Food Leaving an Alkaline Ash

Almonds	Melons
Apples	Milk
Apricots	Onions
Bananas (Ripe)	Oranges
Beets	Parsley

Cabbage	Peaches
Carrots	Pears
Cauliflower	Pineapple
Celery	Potatoes
Coconuts	Pumpkins
Cottage Cheese	Radishes
Cucumbers	Raisins
Dates	Spinach
Figs (Fresh and Dry)	Soyabeans
Grapes	Tomatoes
Lemons	Turnips
Lettuce	
Food Groups	

Food Combining Chart

Food Groups	Proteins	Fats	Starches	Vegetabes	Sweet Fruits	Sub-acid Fruits	Acid Fruits
Proteins	Good	Poor	Poor	Good	Poor	Fair	Good
Fats	Poor	Good	Fair	Good	Fair	Fair	Fair
Starches	Poor	Fair	Good	Good	Fair	Fair	Poor
Vegetable	Good	Good	Good	Good	Poor	Poor	Poor
Sweet Fruits	Poor	Fair	Fair	Poor	Good	Good	Poor
Sub-acid Fruits	Fair	Fair	Fair	Poor	Good	Good	Good
Acid Fruits	Good	Fair	Poor	Poor	Poor	Good	Good

Proteins: Nuts, seeds, soyabeans, cheese, eggs, poultry* meat* fish* yoghurt.

Fats: Oils, olives, butter, margarine.

Starches: Whole cereals, peas, beans, lentils.

Vegetables: Leafy green vegetables, sprouted seeds, cabbage, cauliflower, broccoli, green peas, celery, tomatoes, onions.

Sweet Fruits: Bananas, figs, custard apple, all-dried fruits, dates.

Sub-acid Fruits: Grapes, Pears, apples, peaches, apricots, plums, guavas, raspberries.

Acid Fruits: Grapefruit, lemons, oranges, limes, pineapple, strawberries.

---

* Not recommended for good nutrition

Nature Cure Treatments
(Prescribed in Various Chapters)

(1) Enema

An enema involves the injection of fluid into the rectum. An enema can is required for this purpose. This should be filled with water at 98°F temperature and placed on a suitable hook at a height of four to six feet from the ground. The patient is made to lie on his right side extending his right leg and folding the left leg at right angle. The enema nozzle, lubricated with oil or vaseline, is inserted in the rectum. The water is now allowed to enter into the rectum. Generally, one to two litres of water is injected. The patient may either lie down on his back or walk a little while retaining the water. After five to 10 minutes, the water can be ejected along with the accumulated morbid matter.

A warm-water enema helps to clean the rectum of accumulated faecal matter. This is not only the safest system for cleaning the bowels, but it also improves the peristaltic movement of the bowels and thereby relieves constipation.

(2) Dry Friction

Dry friction bath is an excellent method of keeping the skin in order. It increases the activity of all the functional processes lying at or near the surface of the body. This bath can be taken with a rough dry towel or with a moderately soft bristle brush. If the brush is used, the procedure is as follows. Take the brush in one hand and begin with the face, neck and chest. Then brush one arm, beginning at the wrist and brushing towards the shoulders. Now brush one foot, then the ankle and chest. Then do the other foot and leg, and next the hips and central portion of the body. Continue brushing each part until the skin is pink. Use the brush quickly back and forward on every part of the body. If a towel is used, it should be fairly rough, and the same process gone through as for the use of brush.

(3) Sponge Bath

For giving sponge bath, water should be taken at the required temperature in a basin. The sponge bath may be given either with a turkish towel or with gloves prepared with the turkish cloth. Generally the sponge bath is given to bed-ridden patients who are very weak and to those suffering from prolonged fever or illness. The patient should be covered with a bedsheet and the limbs rubbed one after the other with the turkish towel dipped frequently in water. Soon after the friction, the legs should be dried. The patient should again be covered with the bed sheet. Sponge one part at a time in the following order; arms, chest, abdomen, legs, feet and back. For the arm or leg, spread the towel under the whole length of the arm or leg while it is being sponged. Rub skin briefly with the face towel to draw blood on the surface. Dry each part after the sponge to avoid chilling. Be sure the patient is dry before replacing clothing and covers. In case of very weak patients warm water should be used and for other persons cold water can be used.

(4) Cold Compress

This is a local application using a cloth which has been wrung out in cold water. The cloth should be folded into a broad strip and dipped in cold water or ice water. The compress is generally applied to the head, neck, chest, abdomen and back. The cold compress is an effective indirect means of controlling inflammatory conditions of the liver, spleen, stomach, kidneys, intestines, lungs, brain, pelvic organs and so on.

(5) Wet Pack or Heating Compress

This is a cold compress covered in such a manner as to bring warmth. A heating compress consists of three or four folds of linen cloth wrung out in cold water which is then covered completely with dry flannel or blanket to prevent the circulation or air and help accumulation of body heat. It is sometimes applied for several hours. The duration of the application is determined by the extent and location of the surface involved, the nature and thickness of the coverings and the water temperature. After removing the compress, the area should be rubbed with a wet cloth and dried with a towel. A heating compress can be applied to the throat, chest, abdomen and joints. A throat compress relieves sore throat, hoarseness, tonsillitis, pharyngitis and laryngitis. An abdominal compress helps those suffering from gastritis, hyperacidity, indigestion, jaundice, constipation, diarrhoea, dysentery and other ailments relating to the abdominal organs. The chest compress, also known as chest pack, relieves cold, bronchitis, pleurisy, pneumonia, fever, cough and so on, while the joints compress is helpful for inflamed joints, rheumatism, rheumatic fever and sprains.

(6) Hip Baths

The hip bath is one of the most useful forms of hydrotherapy. As the name suggests, this mode of treatment involves only the hips and the abdominal region below the navel. A special type of tub is used for the purpose. The tub is filled with water in a way that it covers the hips and reaches upto the navel when the patient sits in it. Generally four to six gallons of water is required. If the special tub is not available, a common tub may be used. A support may be placed under one edge to elevate it by two or three inches. Hip bath is given in cold, hot, neutral or alternate temperatures.

(i) Cold Hip Bath

The water temperature should be 10°C to 18°C. The duration of the bath is usually 10 minutes. If the patient feels cold or is very weak, a hot foot immersion should be given with the cold hip bath. The legs should be so adjusted that there is no pressure upon the muscles, ligaments and blood vessels of the knee region.

The patient should rub the abdomen briskly from the naval downwards and across the body with a moderately coarse wet cloth. The legs, feet and upper part of the body should remain completely dry during and after the bath. The patient should undertake moderate exercise after the cold hip bath to warm the body. A cold hip bath is a routine treatment in most diseases. It relieves constipation, indigestion, obesity and helps the eliminative organs to function properly.

(ii) Hot Hip Bath

This bath is generally taken for eight to 10 minutes at a water temperature of 40°C to 45°C. The bath should start at 40°C. The temperature should be gradually increased to 45°C. No friction should be applied to the abdomen. Before entering the tub, the patient should drink one glass of cold water. A cold compress should be placed on the head. Care should be taken to prevent the patient from catching a chill after the bath. The bath should be terminated and the patient should be given a cold shower. A hot hip bath helps to relieve pain in the pelvic organs, painful urination and inflammed rectum or bladder.

(iii) Neutral Hip Bath

The temperature of the water should be 32°C to 36°C. Here too, friction to the abdomen should be avoided. This bath is generally taken for 20 minutes to an hour. The neutral hip bath helps to relieve all acute and sub-acute inflammatory conditions.

(iv) Alternate Hip Bath

This is also known as revulsive hip bath. The temperature in the hot tub should be 40°C to 45°C and in the cold tub 10°C to 18°C . The patient should alternately sit in the hot tub for five minutes and then in the cold tub for three minutes. The duration of the bath is generally 10 to 20 minutes. The head and neck should be kept cold with a cold compress. The treatment should end with a dash of cold water to the hips. The bath relieves chronic inflammatory conditions of the pelvic viscera.

(7) Full Wet Sheet Pack

This is a procedure in which the whole body is wrapped in a wet sheet, which in turn is wrapped in a dry blanket for regulating evaporation. The blanket should be spread on the bed with its edges hanging over the edge of the bed. The upper end should be about eight inches from the head of the bed. Then spread a linen sheet wrung out in cold water over the blanket so that its end is slightly below the upper end of the blanket. The patient should lie on the bedsheet with his shoulders about three inches below the upper edge. The wet sheet should be quickly wrapped round the body of the patient, drawn in, tightly tucked between the legs and also between the body and the arms. The sheet should be folded over the shoulders and across the neck. Now the blanket should be drawn tightly around the body and tucked in along the side in a similar manner, pulling it tightly. The ends should be doubled up at the feet. A turkish towel should be placed below the chin to protect the face and neck from coming into contact with the blanket and to exclude outside air more effectively. The head should be covered with a wet cloth so that the scalp remains cold. The feet should be kept warm during the entire treatment. If the patient's feet are cold, place hot water bottles near them to hasten reaction. The pack is administered for half an hour to one hour to one hour till the patient begins to perspire profusely. He may be given cold or hot water to drink.

This pack is useful in cases of fever, especially in typhoid and continued fevers, and benefits those suffering from insomnia, epilepsy and infantile convulsion. It is useful in relieving chronic cold and bronchitis.

(8) Hot Foot Bath

In this method, the patient should keep his or her legs in a tub or bucket filled with hot water at a temperature of 40°C to 45°C. Before taking the bath a glass of water should be taken and the body should be covered with a blanket so that no heat or vapour escapes from the foot bath. The head should be protected with a cold compress. The duration of the bath is generally from five to 20 minutes. The patient should take a cold shower immediately after the bath. The hot foot bath stimulates the involuntary muscles of the uterus, intestine, bladder and other pelvic and abdominal organs.

(9) Steam Bath

Steam bath is one of the most important time-tested water treatments which induces perspiration in a most natural way. The patient, clad in minimum loin cloth or underwear, is made to sit on a stool inside a specially designed cabinet.

Before entering the cabinet, the patient should drink one or two glasses of cold water and protect the head with a cold towel. The duration of the steam bath is generally 10 to 20 minutes or until profuse perspiration takes place. A cold shower should be taken immediately after the bath.

If the patient feels giddy or uneasy during the steam bath, he or she should immediately be taken out and given a glass of cold water and the face washed with cold water.

The steam bath helps to eliminate morbid matter from the surface of the skin. It also improves circulation of blood and tissue activity. It relieves rheumatism, gout, uric acid problems, jaundice and obesity. The steam bath is helpful in all forms of chronic toxemias. It also relieves neuralgias, chronic nephritis, infections, tetanus and migraine.

(10) Neutral Immersion Bath

This is also known as full bath. It is administered in a bath tub which should be properly fitted with hot and cold water connections. This bath can be given from 15 to 60 minutes at a temperature ranging from 26°C to 28°C. It can be given for long duration, without any ill-effects, as the water temperature is akin to the body temperature. The neutral bath diminishes the pulse rate without modifying respiration. This treatment is the best sedative. Since the neutral bath excites activity of both the skin and the kidneys.

(11) Epsom-Salt Bath

The ordinary bath tub should be filled with about 135 litres of hot water at 40°C. One to one and a half kg of Epsom salt should be dissolved in this water. The patient should drink a glass of cold water, cover the head with a cold towel and then lie down in the tub, completely immersing the trunk, thighs and legs for 15 to 20 minutes. The best time to take this bath is just before retiring to bed. This is useful in cases of sciatica, lumbago, rheumatism, diabetes, neuritis, cold and catarrh, kidney disorders and other uric acid and skin infections.

(12) Spinal Bath

The spinal bath is an important form of hydrotherapic treatment. This bath provides a soothing effect to the spinal column and thereby influences the central nervous system. It is given in a specially designed tub with its back raised so as to provide proper support to the head. The bath can be administered at cold, neutral and hot temperatures. The water level in the tub should be an inch and a half to two inches and the patient should lie in it for 3 to 10 minutes.

The cold spinal bath relieves irritation, fatigue, hypertension and excitement. It is beneficial in almost all nervous disorders, loss of memory and tension. The neutral spinal bath is a soothing and sedative treatment, especially for the highly strung and irritable patient. It is the ideal treatment for insomnia and also relieves tension of the vertebral column. The duration of this bath is 20 to 30 minutes. The hot spinal bath, on the other hand, helps to stimulate the nerves, especially when they are in a depressed state. It also relieves vertebral pain in spondylitis and muscular backache. It relieves sciatic pain and gastrointestinal pain of gastric origin.

(13) Hot Fomentation

A fomentation is a local application of moist heat by means of cloths wrung from hot water. Select a piece of blanket or fannel large enough to fit over the chest or back. Fold it into a pack, dip it in very hot water, and wring it out as dry as possible. Wrap this in a dry Turkish towel, or other material thick enough to protect the skin, and apply the whole pack to the area to be treated. Leave the hot pack in place for ten or fifteen minutes, or until it is cool. Then rub the area with a small piece of ice or a cold cloth and dry the skin with a rough Turkish towel. The fomentation may be reapplied several times, as desired. Follow this with some massage or heavy rubbing. If you are treating a patient with a chest cold, first apply the fomentation to the back, and then later treat the chest. Better still, use two packs at the same time, front and back.

Hot fomentations are useful in treating local pains and muscle injuries in the arms, legs and back. They are also of value in treating chest colds, influenza, cough, bronchitis, laryngitis, pleurisy; and inflammation in any part of the body. Patients suffering from arthritis can also benefit from this treatment. However, the greatest value of this form of water treatment is found in cases of colds and respiratory infection.

(14) Sun Bath

Sun bath consists of the application of natural sunlight directly to the exposed body surface. Sun bath should be taken between

8 a.m. and 11 a.m. and between 2 p.m. and 4 p.m. in summer between 7 a.m. and 9 a.m. and between 3 p.m. and 5 p.m. The sun bath can be taken by exposing either the whole or a part of the body to the direct exposure of the solar rays. The patient should commence the treatment for 5 minutes on the 1st day. The duration should be gradually increased by 5 minutes daily to 2 to 3 hours in the final stage. The head should not be exposed and the eyes should be protected against glare by shielding them with coloured glasses or a dark cloth. In the alternative, cold wet compresses may be used to cover the head and the eyes. The patient should drink a glass of cold water before starting the bath and also drink water whenever he feels thirsty during the bath. The treatment should be concluded by cooling douche or wet hand rub so as to cool and invigorate the skin.

Sunlight promotes health and prevents disease. The direct rays of the sun kill disease germs in a very short time. Maximum results can be attained if sunshine can be made to fall directly upon the diseased tissues. This bath also vitalizes and energizes the body and increases its resistance power.

(15) Mud Packs

The use of mud packs has been found highly beneficial and effective in the treatment of chronic inflammations caused by internal diseases, bruises, sprains, boils and wounds. A mud pack is prepared with clay obtained from about ten cms, below the surface of the earth, after ensuring that it does not contain any impurities such as compost or pebbles. The clay is then made into a smooth paste with warm water. This is allowed to cool and then spread on a strip or cloth, the size of which may vary according to requirements. The dimensions of the pack meant for application on the abdomen are generally 20 cms × 10 cms × 2.5 cms for adults. As the abdomen is the seat of most diseases, mud pack applied to this part of the body can cure many disorders including all forms of indigestion affecting the stomach and bowels. It is most effective in decreasing the external heat and breaking up the morbid matter.

(16) Massage

Massage is an excellent form of passive exercise. It involves the scientific manipulation of the soft tissues of the body. If correctly done on a bare body, it can be highly stimulating and invigorating. The general massage, dealing with all parts of the body, tones up the nervous system, influences respiration and quickens the elimination of poisons and waste material from the body through the various eliminative organs such as lungs, skin, kidneys and bowels. It also boosts blood circulation and metabolic processes.

Cotton seed oil is most commonly used for massaging. If the patient is averse to oil, talcum powder may be used. General body massage may be done for 40 to 45 minutes and local body massage for 10 to 15 minutes. The oil should be washed off completely after massage.

(i) Abdominal Massage

This form of massage is beneficial in constipation. It stimulates the peristalsis of the small intestines, tones up the muscles of the abdomen walls and mechanically eliminates the contents of both large and small intestines. Abdominal massage should not be done after a heavy meal, but after two hours or so. The bladder should be emptied before the massage. The patient is made to lie on his back with his knees drawn up. This enables the abdomen wall to relax. The massuer should stand at the right side of the patient and use finger tips for friction round the umbilical region from right to left. He should likewise alternatively knead the walls and roll with both hands, making deep and firm pressure. He should knead with heel of the hand and finger tips and later take up massaging the larger intestines. The manipulation of the large intestine should begin on the right side. Keep it going upwards and across the transverse colon and move right down on the left side to the sigmoid flexure and rectum. Circular kneading should be done with the help of the three middle fingers. At the same time, press into the contents of the abdomen, following the course of the larger colon with a crawling motion. Keep kneading by means of a few circular movements in one spot with the help of finger tips. Keep moving the fingers a little further along. Knead repeatedly. Use knuckles of the hand to make deep pressures along the larger colon, moving the hands along after each pressure.

(ii) Chest Massage

Chest massage strengthens the chest muscles, increases circulation and tones up the nervous system of the chest, heart and lungs. It is especially recommended in weakness of the lungs, palpitation and organic heart disorders.

The patient is made to lie on the back with the arms at the sides. The masseur starts manipulating the chest by means of strokes with both hands on each side of the breast bone. A circular motion is formed by the movement made up and down, moving down the chest. Next the muscle kneading is done by picking up the skin and muscles with both hands. Treatment is given on both the sides of the chest likewise. Circular kneading is next done by placing one hand on each side of the breast bone and making the circular motions outward towards the sides.

(iii) Massage of the Throat

This helps to overcome headache, sore throat and catarrh of the throat. The patient is made to throw his head back. The masseur places palms of both hands on neck with thumbs under the chin, and fingers under the ears. A downward stroke is next made towards the chest over the jugular veins. Do not exert heavily on the jugular veins. Repeat several times.

(17) Yogic Kriyas

A disease-free system should be the starting ground for yogasanas and pranayama. There are six specific cleaning techniques, known as Shat Kriyas, which eliminate impurities and help cure many ailments. Of these, the following three can be practised by older children safely.

(i) Jalaneti

Jalaneti is a process of cleansing the air passage of the nostrils and the throat by washing them with tepid saline water. Take a clean jalaneti pot. Put half a teaspoonful of salt in the pot and fill it with lukewarm drinking water.

Stand up and tilt your head slightly to the right. Insert the nozzle of the pot in the left nostril and let the water flow into it. Inhale and exhale through the mouth, allowing the water to flow out through the right nostril. Reverse this process by tilting your head to the left and letting the water flow from the right to the left nostril.

Jalaneti should be practised only in the morning. It will relieve sore throat, cold, cough, sinusitis, migraine, headache and cases of inflammation of the nasal membranes. It keeps the head cool and improves vision.

(ii) Kunjal or Vamana Dhouti

This is a process of cleansing the interior of the stomach. Drink four to six glasses of tepid water with a little salt added to it early in the morning on an empty stomach. Then stand up, bend forward, insert the middle and index fingers of the right hand into the mouth until they touch the uvula. Tickle it until you feel a vomiting sensation. The saline water thus ejected will bring up bile and other toxic matter with it. Repeat the process till all the water is vomited out. This should be done once a week or as and when necessary. It is beneficial for cleansing the stomach in cases of excessive bile, constipation and gastric troubles.

(iii) Kapalabhati

This is a respiratory exercise for the abdomen and diaphragm. The channels inside the nose and other parts of the respiratory system are purified by this exercise. In the process, the brain is also cleared. Sit in a comfortable position, preferably in padmasana. Exercise the diaphragm by exhaling suddenly and quickly through both nostrils, producing a hissing sound. Inhaling will be automatic and passive. The air should be exhaled from the lungs with a sudden, vigorous inward stroke of the front abdominal muscles. The abdominal stroke should be completed and the breath should be expelled fully. While inhaling, no willful expansion is necessary and the abdominal muscles should be relaxed. This exercise should be done in three phases, each consisting of 20 to 30 strokes a minute. A little rest can be taken in between. Throughout, the thoracic muscles should be kept contracted. Kapalabhati enables the inhalation of a good amount of oxygen which purifies the blood and strengthens the nerve and brain centres. This kriya provides relief in many lung, throat and chest diseases like chronic bronchitis, asthma, pleurisy and tuberculosis.

(18) Pranayama

(i) Anuloma-viloma

Sit in any comfortable meditative pose, keeping your head, neck and spine erect. Rest your left hand on your left knee. Close your right nostril by pressing the tip of your right thumb against it. Breathe out slowly through the left nostril. Inhale slowly and deeply through the left nostril, keeping the right nostril closed. Close your left nostril with the little finger and ring finger of your right hand and exhale through the right nostril, keeping the left nostril closed and lastly, exhale through the left nostril, keeping the right nostril closed. This completes one round of anuloma-viloma. Repeat the entire process. Inhaling and exhaling should be done very slowly, without making any sound. This pranayama is a process of purification. It strengthens the lungs and calms the nerves. It helps cure cough and cold, insomnia, chronic headache and asthma.

(ii) Ujjayi

Sit in any comfortable meditative pose. Inhale slowly, deeply and steadily through both nostrils with a low uniform sound through the glottis. Hold your breath for a second or two after inhaling and then exhale noisily only through the left nostril, keeping the right nostril closed. Do this as often as required. This pranayama clears the nasal passage and helps the functioning of the thyroid gland and benefits respiratory disorders, especially bronchitis and asthma.

(iii) Bhramari

In this pranayama, the buzzing sound of a bee is produced and hence it is called bhramari. Keep your mouth closed while inhaling. Exhale through both nostrils, producing the humming sound of a bee. This pranayama affects the ears, nose, eyes and mouth and makes the complexion glow. It also helps those suffering from insomnia.

Glossary

Abdomen: The part of the body between the chest and the pelvis containing the digestive organs.

Abscess: Localised collection of pus in the body tissues.

Absorption: The process by which digested foods from the intestine enter into the blood or lymph.

Acidosis: A condition in which the acidity of body fluid is abnormally high.

Acute: Any process which has sudden onset and runs a relatively severe and short course.

Addiction: Habituation to certain drugs, foods or drinks.

Adrenaline: A hormone secreted by the central part of the adrenal glands.

Adhesion: Abnormal growing together of tissues, usually after inflammation or injury.

Adolescence: The period of growth from 13 to 18 years of age.

Ageing: The process or the effects of growing mature or old.

Albumin: A protein substance found in all living organisms.

Allergy: Sensitivity of an individual to certain substances which do not affect most other people.

Allergen: A substance capable of producing allergy.

Alleviate: Relief from symptoms.

Alveoli: Air containing vesicles.

Amino acids: Chemical compounds out of which proteins are formed.

Amoeba: A microscopic animal consisting of one single cell.

Anaemia: Deficiency of red blood cells.

Androgen: A male sex hormone.

Analgesic: A drug for relieving pain.

Aneurysm: Dilation of the artery due to weakened wall.

Angina Pectoris: A pain in the chest caused by diminished supply of blood to the heart.

Ankylosis: Stiffness of a joint.

Antibiotic: A chemical substance having the power to retard the growth of certain germs.

Antibody: Substances capable of counteracting the bacteria or bacterial products.

Antidote: A substance used to counteract effect of poison or disease.

Antigen: A protein which induces a reaction in the body and produces antibodies.

Antioxidant: A substance that has the ability to prevent or delay deterioration caused by the oxygen.

Antiseptic: A substance which inhibits the growth of or destroys micro organisms.

Antispasmodic: Drugs relaxing the contracted muscles.

Antitoxin: Substance formed in the blood stream, capable of combating certain poisons within the body.

Anus: Outlet of alimentary canal.

Aorta: The main artery of the body.

Appendicitis: Inflammation of the vermiform appendix.

Apoplexy: Brain haemorrhage or stroke.

Arteriosclerosis: A condition of loss of elasticity and thickening of coats of the arteries with inflammatory changes.

Arthritis: Painful swelling of joints.

Atrophy: Wasting of the tissues.

Atherosclerosis: Hardening of the arteries.

Atrium: Auricle or upper chamber of the heart.

Aura: A sensation occurring prior to the onset of an epileptic fit.

Autonomic System: The part of the nervous system which controls the vital organs, and which is involuntary.

Bacillus: A rod-shaped bacteria.

Bacteria: Microbe, micro-organism.

Benign: Tumour or condition which is not malignant or cancerous.

Barium: An opaque chemical compound for visualising the gastrointestinal tract under X-ray.

Bile: A greenish-brown fluid secreted by the liver.

Biopsy: Removal of a piece of tissue from the patient for the purpose of gross and microscopic examination to diagnose a disease.

Black out: Fainting.

Blood count: Calculation of number of red or white blood cells in a cubic millimeter of blood.

Boil: A painful abscess at the hair root.

Bowel: Intestine, often applied to large intestine.

Bronchiectasis: Dilation of the bronchi, the air passages.

Bronchiole: Tiny branches of the bronchus.

Bronchus: Branches of windpipe.

Bunion: A swelling of the main joint of the great toe.

Caecum: A blind sac at the junction of the small and large intestines.

Calcification: A process by which organic tissue becomes hardened by disposition of calcium salts within its substance.

Calculus: A stone or stony mass of minerals formed within the body.

Calorie: Unit of heat used for measuring the energy value of food.

Capillary: A tiny blood-vessel, connecting a vein and artery.

Cancer: Uncontrolled devastating growth of cells.

Carbohydrate: Starchy food which furnishes energy.

Carcinogen: Any substance capable of causing cancer.

Carcinoma: Malignant or cancerous tumour of the skin or internal organs.

Cardiac: Pertaining to the heart.

Cerebral: Related to the brain.

Cervical spine: The top portion of the spine (neck), composed of seven vertebrae.

Cholesterol: A yellowish fatty substance synthesized in the liver and supplied in the diet.

Chronic: Long continuous course of disease.

Cirrhosis: Fibrous scar replacing the cells.

Coma: An unconscious state from which the patient cannot be aroused.

Complication: A condition developing during disease process.

Congenital: A condition existing from birth.

Constipation: Difficult or infrequent bowel movements.

Convalescence: Gradual recovery from illness.

Convulsions: A violent and involuntary contraction or series of contractions of the voluntary muscles.

Cornea: The transparent circular portion of the front of the eyeball.

Coronary: Arteries supplying blood to the heart muscles that encircle the heart like a crown.

Coronary thrombosis: A blockage of the blood flow caused by a blood clot in a coronary artery.

Cortisone: A steroid hormone secreted by the outer part of the adrenal glands.

Cramp: Sharp muscular pain.

Cystitis: Inflammation of the urinary bladder.

Decoction: A process of boiling down so as to extract some essence.

Dehydration: Abnormal loss of body fluids.

Delirium: A state of mental confusion and excitement.

Diagnosis: Identification of disease by patient's symptoms and other methods.

Diaphragm: Muscle separating chest from abdomen.

Diastolic: Lower level of the blood pressure within the arteries when the heart is at rest

Dimentia: Loss of intellectual function.

Disease: The abnormal functioning of the body organ.

Disinfection: Process of destroying pathogenic or harmful microorganisms.

Diverticulosis: Abnormal pockets or pouches within a mucous membrane of the colon.

Douche: Washing with a stream of water.

Dropsy: Accumulation of water in tissues

Ductless Glands: Glands which pour their secretions directly into the blood stream without benefit of a connecting tube.

Duodenum: First part of the small intestine adjacent to stomach.

Electrocardiograph: Diagnostic instrument used to record the electrical currents generated in the heart.

Embolus: A foreign body which forms an obstruction in the blood vessel.

Emphysema: Abnormal presence of gas or air in the body tissues. Widening of air sacs in the lungs.

Endemic: Disease prevalent in a particular area.

Endocardium: A tough glistening membrane which lines the four chambers of the heart.

Endocrine: Glands secreting hormones.

Enema: Injection of water or other liquid into the colon via the anus.

Estrogen: One of two hormones secreted by the ovaries.

Enzymes: Complex organic substances secreted by living cells, important in digestion and other bodily functions.

Epilepsy: A chronic disease usually functional, charectarised by brief convulsive seizures and loss of consciousness.

Excretion: Removal of wastes from the body.

Expectoration: The act of coughing up and spitting out materials from the lungs and trachea.

Expiration: Process of breathing out.

Fatty acids: One of the end products of fat digestion.

Fissure: A crack in the membrane lining the rectum.

Flatulence: Distension of the stomach or intestines with air of gases.

Follicle: A pocket in the dermis containing a hair root.

Fomentation: A hot, moist pack or application to the body.

Gangrene: Localised death of tissues.

Gastric: Pertaining to the stomach.

Gene: Hereditary factor present in all cells.

Geriatrics: The branch of medicine that deals with the structural changes, physiology, diseases and hygiene of old age.

Gerontology: The scientific study of the process and phenomena of ageing.

Gland: An organ that produces a specific secretion.

Globulin: A blood protein which contains antibodies.

Glottis: The opening of windpipe.

Glutanic acid: A naturally occurring amino acid, a constituent of many proteins.

Goitre: Enlargement of thyroid.

Gonads: Testicles and ovaries.

Gynaecology: Medical science dealing with the treatment of disorders of female reproductive system.

Haemoglobin: Oxygen-carrying pigment found in red blood cells.

Hallucination: A mental impression having no foundation in fact.

Hay fever: Seasonal allergic reaction to pollen.

Heartburn: Burning sensation in upper abdomen and chest.

Hepatitis: Inflammation of the liver.

Heredity: The transmission of traits from parents to offspring.

Hernia: Rupture or protrusion of organ or part of an organ through the wall of a body cavity.

Hormone: A glandular secretion that regulates body functions.

Hyperacidity: An excessive degree of acidity.

Hypertension: Increased level of blood pressure.

Ileum: Terminal portion of the small intestine.

Immunity: Capacity of the body to resist infection.

Impotence: Inability to have an erection.

Infarction: death of tissue due to interruption of its blood supply.

Infection: Invasion of the body by microorganisms.

Infestation: The invasion of the body by parasites.

Inflammation: A reaction of the body tissues to injury, infection or irritation.

Ingestion: The act of taking food, medicines, etc., by mouth.

Inhalation: The drawing in of air or other vapour into the lungs.

Insulin: The hormone of the pancreas which controls the blood sugar level.

Insomnia: The inability to sleep

Intercellular: In between the cells.

Jaundice: A yellow colouration of the skin due to excess of bile pigments in the blood.

Lactose: Milk sugar.

Larynx: Voice box.

Laxative: A mild purgative.

Lesion: A localised tissue damage caused by injury or disease.

Leukaemia: A blood disease in which the white blood cells increase enormously in number.

Ligaments: A tough fibrous band connecting bones or other tissues of the body.

Lymph: The clear, liquid part of the blood which enters the spaces between body cells.

Malignant tumour: Cancer with spreading power.

Marrow: The soft tissue in the hollow spaces of the bones.

Mastication: Chewing.

Membrane: A thin tissue serving to line or cover an organ.

Metabolism: The sum of the body processes involving the building up and breaking down of tissues.

Micturition: Process of passing urine.

Mucilage: A sticky substance extracted from certain plants.

Mucus: Lubricating fluid secreted by the mucous membranes of the body.

Mucous membrane: Smooth, soft lining of the passages and cavities of the body.

Myocardial: Pertaining to the heart muscles.

Myopia: Short sight.

Nausea: Vomiting sensation.

Neuralgia: Pain in a nerve.

Neurone: Nerve cell.

Neurosis: Emotional disorder caused by some inner conflict.

Node: A knot or swelling.

Nutrient: A food substance.

Rash: A temporary eruption on the skin.

Rectum: Lower end of the large intestine.

Relapse: Recurrence of symptoms.

Respiration: Process of breathing

Response: A reaction to a stimulus.

Retina: Light sensitive area at the back of the eye.

Sclerosis: Hardening of the tissues.

Screening: Testing, viewing with x-ray under a fluorescent screen.

Sebaceous glands: Glands secreting and conveying oily matter to lubricate the skin or hair.

Secretion: A product of the activity of a gland.

Sedative: A drug or a substance which reduces excitement, irritation and pain.

Senility: The mental and physical weakness of old age.

Serum: The clear portion of blood separated from its clot.

Sinuses: Hollow cavities in the nasal bones.

Skimmed milk: Milk from which cream has been removed.

Sphygmomanometer: An instrument that measures blood pressure.

Sprain: Injury to the ligament surrounding the joint.

Sputum: Material coughed up from the lungs.

Stimulant: Producing rapid transient increase of vital energy in organism or some part of it.

Stool: A faecal discharge from the bowels.

Stroke: A cerebral haermorrhage or bleeding in the brain. A sudden and severe attack as of paralysis.

Susceptibility: Liability to get a disease; opposite of immunity.

Syndrome: A set of signs and symptoms occurring together as an expression of a disorder of function.

Systolic: Upper level of the blood pressure indicating the greatest force exerted by the heart.

Tendon: A tough strand which attaches a muscle to a bone.

Thrombosis: Clogging of a blood-vessel caused by the formation of a clot.

Thyrotoxicosis: Overactivity of the thyroid gland.

Toxin: A poisonous substance produced by the action of microorganisms.

Trachea: Windpipe.

Tranquillizer: Drug used to quieten the nerves.

Trauma: Injury.

Tumour: Abnormal growth of a mass of cells in the body.

Ulcer: An open sore on the skin.

Uraemia: A morbid condition due to the excessive presence of urinary matter in the blood.

Ureter: Duct carrying urine from the kidney to the bladder.

Urethra: Duct carrying urine from the bladder to the exterior.

Uric Acid: A normal constituent of blood and urine metabolism.

Vagina: Female genital passage.

Varicose: Dilated tortuous veins.

Ventilation: Continuous supply of fresh air.

Vesicle: A small sac containing liquid.

Vital: Essential to life.

Wheezing: Noisy and difficult breathing usually due to bronchial asthma.

Bibliography

(1) Exton-Smith A Norman and Weksler Marc E, *Practical Geriatric Medicine*, 1985, Churchill Livingstone, Edinburgh.

(2) Carper Jean, Foods — *Your Miracle Medicine*, 1995, Simon and Schuster, London.

(3) Bakhru H.K., *A Complete Handbook of Nature Cure*, Second edition, fifth impression, 1996, Jaico Publishing House, Mumbai.

(4) Bakhru H.K., *Natural Home Remedies for Common Ailments*, second printing 1996, Orient Paperbacks, Delhi.

(5) Smith A.N., *Metabolic and Nutritional Disorders in the Elderly* 1980, John Wright and Sons Ltd., Bristol.

(6) Anderson R. Clifford, *Your Guide to Health*, seventh edition 1979, Oriental Watchman Publishing House, Pune.

(7) Hodkinson H.M., *An Outline of Geriatrics*, second edition 1981. Academic Press, London.

(8) Wasir H.S., *Ageing and Heart Care*, 1993, Vikas Publishing House Pvt. Ltd., Delhi.

(9) Airola Paavo, *How To Get Well.* 18th printing 1982, Health Plus Publishers, Arizona.

(10) Benjamin Harry, *Everybody's Guide to Nature Care*, second impression 1983, Thorsons Publishers Ltd., Wellingborough.

(11) Singh S.J., *Baths*, second revised edition 1978, Nature Cure Research Hospital, Lucknow.

(12) Sauessele Herman P., *Health and Vigor after Forty with Natural Foods and Vitamins*, 1965, Arco Publishing Co., New York.

(13) Clark Linda, *Stay Young Longer*, fourth printing 1981, Jove Publications, New York.

(14) Kordel Lelord, *How to Keep Your Youthful Vitality After Forty*. Award Books.

(15) Editorial Committee of Science of Life Books. *Live Longer And Healthier*, Third impression 1978, Science of Life Books, Melbourne, Victoria.

Index

www.ingramcontent.com/pod-product-compliance
Ingram Content Group UK Ltd.
Pitfield, Milton Keynes, MK11 3LW, UK
UKHW021709190726
13853UKWH00001B/479

9 788172 246297